The Light Around the Dark

The Light Around the Dark

Elizabeth D. Gee

Formerly Interim Executive Director
The University of Colorado Center for Human Caring

Center for Human Caring

National League for Nursing Press • New York
Pub. No. 14-2476

The Center for Human Caring

The Center for Human Caring was established in 1986 by the University of Colorado School of Nursing. The Center is the nation's first interdisciplinary center with an overall commitment to develop and use knowledge of human caring and healing as the foundation for a dramatically new health care system—a system that affirms and sustains human caring and healing activities as both the moral and scientific basis of clinical practice.

The Center's overall mission is to explore new ways of advancing the art and science of human caring knowledge, ethics and clinical practice in the fields of nursing and health sciences. The Center activities seek to re-establish the critical balance between traditional biomedical technology and human caring by drawing upon the underdeveloped connections between nursing science, caring theory, philosophy, and knowledge from the humanities.

Center efforts range from focused academic-curricular activities, to piloting and researching new educational and clinical practice models of caring excellence.

The Center offers public and professional forums and institutes. It offers formal coursework for credit or non-credit. The Center hosts resident scholars from the humanities and from other diverse academic backgrounds.

The Center provides a forum for interdisciplinary and international dialogue, formal education and research between and among educators, scientists, practitioners, artists, government experts, policy makers and the public.

Human caring knowledge and information is disseminated through formal conferences, sponsored programs and publications. Most of the official Center publications are published and distributed by the National League for Nursing Press in New York.

This book was set in Goudy by Publications Development Company. The editor and designer was Allan Graubard. Northeastern Press was the printer and binder. The cover was designed by Lillian Welsh.

Printed in the United States of America

For Rebekah, Gordon
and
William A. Robinson, MD, PhD

❧ *Through a Lyrical Lens*

Prelude   The introduction; a preparation; the overture.

Scherzo   A momentary relief; life's riddle.

Etude   Elizabeth Gee's view of her experience; and a lens through which we may "study" Elizabeth and her experience.

Intermezzo A short, independent composition; the piece between.

Coda   A concluding passage formally distinct from the main structure.

ও Contents

Prelude

The *Light Around the Dark,* by Elizabeth D. Gee, is more than an official Center for Human Caring publication. This publication is unique in that Elizabeth D. Gee was instrumental in the establishment of the Center as a formal entity at the University of Colorado in the mid 1980s. During the time of its founding, from 1985 to 1987, Dr. Elizabeth D. Gee was the first interim director of the Center. She also held appointments as a lecturer and adjunct assistant professor in the School of Nursing until 1990. In addition, she served as an active member of the Visiting Board of the University of Colorado School of Nursing/Center for Human Caring from 1988 until her death.

Dr. Gee died at her home in Ohio on December 17, 1991. She was 46 years old. She had been battling a recurrence of breast cancer that was diagnosed in 1987 when she was at the University of Colorado, where her husband was president; the cancer recurred in March, 1990.

Elizabeth Gee was a nationally recognized expert in medical and legal ethics and the wife of The Ohio State University President E. Gordon Gee and mother of Rebekah Gee. A native of Utah, Dr. Gee received her BA from the University of Utah in 1968, her MA in history from Brigham Young University in 1979, and her EdD in higher education from West Virginia University.

But this information elucidates only objective, biographical data about Elizabeth's education and her position and formal links with nursing, health sciences, and the Center for Human Caring—it provides only the barest circumstances surrounding her life and death.

In 1985, when Gordon and Elizabeth Gee arrived at the University of Colorado, Gordon assumed the presidency of the university; Elizabeth silently and elegantly assumed her personal and professional goals in the university and the state. Soon she was seen and valued in the university and the state as a gift of immeasurable sophistication, intellect, dedication, beauty, and grace of spirit and action.

As wife of a university president, Elizabeth felt very strongly about having her own professional career. Her involvements with the Center for Human Caring and the School of Nursing were her first professional activities upon arrival in Colorado. Her background in higher education, with a special focus in interdisciplinary studies, humanities, and ethics fit perfectly with the Center's goals and objectives.

Elizabeth had an immediate grasp of what I was trying to accomplish through the Center: "to explore new ways of developing and applying the art and science of human caring knowledge, ethics, and clinical practice in nursing and health sciences." She understood and supported the Center's efforts "to foster the study, teaching, and practice of human caring by drawing upon the undeveloped connections between nursing's caring theories and knowledge from the humanities."

Elizabeth was often a silent partner with me in helping to clarify and formalize application of the rapidly growing feminist literature, literary and ethical knowledge, and new scientific understandings linking human caring modalities with health and healing outcomes.

She was pivotal in working with the Center in developing public and professional forums and institutes, hosting resident scholars from diverse backgrounds, sponsoring interdisciplinary programs and disseminating information through formal and informal educational programs and official publications.

This Center publication, *The Light Around the Dark*, details Elizabeth's personal experiences as a cancer patient. Her story begins with an entry dated September 4, 1987, and concludes with the epilogue dated October 9, 1990.

Elizabeth helps us to experience first hand the interplay between the subjectively real—the physical—the metaphysical; the connectedness of the mindbodyspirit; the mundane acts of the days and moments of our existence that become profoundly complicated; the existentially mysterious;—her journal helps us to see some of the light and shadows of life that are knowable and unknowable at the same time.

The Light Around the Dark also tells Elizabeth Gee's inner story of caring, her life of living her ethics and her humanity, her aesthetics. It tells her story of suffering, of triumph, of despair, her refinements and appreciations, her joys and accomplishments. In this work anyone who has been touched by these small, profound, simple, yet extraordinary and subjectively complex experiences associated with cancer will be lit and lifted up by the peace and strength she sought and found through her life. All will be softened and encouraged by her tumultuous, yet victorious struggles with living and dying, with being connected, being alone, mothering, spousing—in being all she could be: a light around the dark and a sweet soul who lingers still.

All who read this work will feel her spirit, which was crystalline—vivid, clear, brilliant and multifaceted to look at and to know—a mirror for all to see and experience—a prism of life's rainbow—a dance of bright multicolored hues of grace, style, beauty, intellect, and good humor. Elizabeth's spirit, energy, love of life, her wit, charm, and unselfish giving will live on.

During my last conversation with Elizabeth, she confided that having her journal published as a Center for Human Caring publication brought her a sense of personal closure—a circular completion to her professional interests and accomplishments during the past six years of her life. I am honored to have been touched by Elizabeth's spirit and life. The Center for Human Caring is endebted to Elizabeth Gee for her gift of light.

I offer my continuing thanks to the National League for Nursing Press for supporting the activities of the Center for Human Caring. I express my deep appreciation to the League for making this special Center for Human Caring publication possible.

Jean Watson, PhD, RN, FAAN
Director of The Center for Human
Caring and Professor of Nursing
University of Colorado Health
Sciences Center

December 26, 1991

Scherzo

❧ *Life's Riddle*

Elizabeth Gee was a scholar in medical ethics, ethics and the law, and women's studies. At once, she was a woman uniquely talented in human relationships: she knew as much as anyone about what being a wife should mean, being a mother, being a friend. Also, she understood things about the natural world and the wonders of the earth—burgeoning in spring, sparkling in summer, glowing gold-red in fall, blanketed in winter, always pulsing somehow, promising new vistas to be felt and seen and explored.

Her intellectual range, her sensitivities, her perceptual acuity: all these fed into the quality of mind that is so evident in these journals. Startling perceptions and insights stud the accounts of her advancing illness; it is as if windows keep opening in winding corridors, windows that disclose sudden colors and shafts of light, colors and lights that illuminate but never for a moment deceive.

She made particularly clear the value of naming, of articulating a personal story, a narrative of what it has meant to be alive. To find words, as Elizabeth Gee has done, is to refuse to be victim. Description itself—especially the delicate, particularized description this writer was capable of—becomes a way of sense-making. Moreover, it becomes a way of leaving a thumb-print on the always unravelling scheme of things, a sign that one was *here*.

From the vantage point of the health professions, these journals may be significant in providing an unusually candid, reflective view of the lived experience of cancer from the perspective of the person living it. Their potency is in part due to the fact that Elizabeth Gee lived for twenty years under the shadow of breast cancer and, without ever denying the threat, created a remarkable and productive life. And the potency is in part due to the clear and unabashed ring of the voice made audible through these pages. Its sounds ring true, painfully true; "life's riddle" remains unsolved. But they are silvery sounds in spite of all. Even as the reader (like the friend) cannot but feel a kind of outrage that such a life had to end so soon, there remain the affirmations of the wonders of existence (and bravery and delight) for Elizabeth Gee and those for whom she left this book. She will be remembered; she will be thanked.

Maxine Greene, PhD
Professor Emeritus
Teachers College,
Columbia University

Etude

ঌ Enter In

Surgery will be in ten days. Gordon, my husband, and Rebekah, our eleven-year-old daughter, and I are spending the Labor Day weekend in our small mountain home in Colorado. We left the city to compose from the news that I will soon have a major operation. We haven't told Rebekah about the surgery, but will tonight. She will be relieved to know what's wrong. Gordon and I have been trying to act normal toward her since we met with the doctors a few days ago, but her eyes shift between us, back and forth, studying our gestures and awkward glances. Occasionally, she says something horrible, just to experiment with our reaction, as if to throw out a line to see if we will bite. Although I know what she is doing, I lose control and snap at her anyway. Gordon's affable disposition that usually expands in the relaxing atmosphere of the mountains seems to be closing in on itself. There is a stiffness in his shoulders which round in like a protective frame. He sits curled up for hours on a bedroom chair, one leg hanging over the arm, head pressed to the upholstery, left hand covering half of his face. He is talking on the phone about university business as though immersion in professional work will carry him to a place where this isn't happening. Flashes of twelve years as the mother of this child and twenty years as the wife of this man stare back at me in the mirror from across a counter cf cold pink tile: little cloth-covered buttons forced through small buttonholes; chubby legs bending to fit into a yellow, flannel sleep suit; the smell of burnt pork roast and a ruined dinner for Gordon's law school classmates; sitting with Gordon on an orange bedspread, eating Mexican TV Dinners.

A week ago I discovered a lump in my breast. This is not the first lump I have found nor my first operation. For twenty years some "mass" has appeared at least every year, requiring observation, a biopsy, or else major surgery. Every time a physician tells me, "you have a small lump," words I have heard dozens of times since my marriage, a quiet madness starts weaving through me like blood-red yarn into a loom. Numbness starts climbing from my chin, up my face to my brain. For a few moments, I can't hear the doctor. His lips round and press together, but there is no sound. Minutes pass before word fragments merge into sentences.

These on and off again health crises have instilled in me a kind of darkness. I feel as though I am in a nightmare, that I am held in the ocean by the pull of an undertow. When I was twelve, I dreamed I was a tiny point on a beach. An enormous wave rose like a mountain above my head. In seconds it would open its mouth, sweeping me into a raging funnel of green water and seaweed. I was frozen. I couldn't move. The beach was empty—no bathers, no surfers, no lifeguard in white trunks, no mother watching from a big green towel anchored on each corner with brown paper grocery bags. I could taste the ocean and feel salty bubbles tighten my breath. The wave rose higher until it seemed the top curls of froth were miles up in the sky. Suddenly I was gone, stamped out of my dream. An overwhelming feeling of nothingness remained that I can still call back to this day. Next I remember sitting up in bed, screaming, and running downstairs to where my mother and grandparents sat around the kitchen table. I tried to speak but was trembling so hard the words would not come. Grandpa Cannon took me into the next room and sat me between the piano and the parlor clock. Then he offered a prayer, a "blessing," to help me stop shaking. I don't know what he said to God, but the torment stopped suddenly.

September 5, 1987

I have had numerous needle aspirations and two surgical biopsies in the last few years, both benign. "Significant fibrocystic disease," they say—meaning the condition in which the breast tends to have numerous benign nodules. A family history of breast cancer apparently increases my risk. I have no sister, but it is present in both sides of my family, my father's line probably carrying the stronger risk: his mother had a mastectomy in her early sixties, and her sister developed cancer in both breasts. One of my two paternal cousins also developed bilateral breast cancer. However, two of my mother's five sisters have also had breast cancer: Florence died of the disease in her twenties, and her older sister, Rachel, now eighty, developed breast cancer a few years ago. For years I have felt this impending threat as if these women are reaching to link hands with mine. Several years back, I started thinking about having a subcutaneous mastectomy, an operation in which most of the breast tissue is removed. I have researched the procedure and consulted with several surgeons. No doctor will guarantee a cancer-free result, yet the consensus is that it is a reasonable option. It might help prevent cancer, or at the very least make further diagnosis more reliable. I told my doctors that I did not want another biopsy. I did not want to be biopsied year after year. Scar tissue might mask a cancer. "Am I foolish to consider a mastectomy?" I asked one doctor. "How dangerous is the surgery?" He rested his hand on my shoulder. "It is a good choice; you'll be fine," he said.

Gordon rinses the plates and props them in the dishwasher. I spray the glass table until bread crumbs float on little pools. There is a richness in these moments now. I imagine thin reefs of stones in the stream by our house. It is almost like seeing for the first time, seeing a simple day, in the pebbles and eddies curling around.

September 6, 1987

How can I speak about my involvement with prayer? Can language express what a soul sees or says? Let me simply say that my spirit engages in heartfelt conversation with God. The process transcends thought, moves past logic, beyond conventional ways of talking and thinking. I may be taken as pretentious, or as a fanatic, but I would like to share this part of my being. It is personal and poignant, a source of much of who I am.

Gordon and I kneel by the bed. The room is dark except for the glimmer of the brass headboard. Gordon starts to speak. His voice is relaxed and calm. Each phrase seems to find an indistinct route across an unseen border.

My Grandmother Cannon, standing by the bedside of her dying mother, listens to her father pray for his wife to die: "Release her. It's time." Grandma can't believe what she hears. "Bless mother to die? No!" She runs outside and screams at God to make her mother well. Then she experiences a peculiar splendor. Words rush through her mind: "In the death of your mother, the will of the Lord has been done." She fills with piercing love. She is so much at peace now that she returns to the house and takes her little brother, Heber, in her arms. "It's OK for Mother to die, Heber. I know now it's right."

She is only twelve. She says nothing for a while. As she grows she finds the courage to tell the story, sometimes at church. But each time she does, a thought comes: "I don't know whether I heard that; I only thought I did."

Then one Sunday when she is twenty-two, her father speaks at church. He tells of his wife's death, how he prayed for her suffering to stop and for her to die. He describes how, as his daughter ran out the back door, he fell to his knees and prayed: "I can stand the death of my wife, but not the loss of my child's faith!" For the first time, she learns of her father's prayer. For the first time, she knows that he prayed for a window to open between her and God.

September 8, 1987

Rebekah is frightened. I can feel her desperation as if she were struck by that great wave in my dream. I see myself at ten standing by my mother when someone on the phone tells her my father is dead.

She is sitting at a card table in the middle of my playroom, sewing something—perhaps doll clothes. Maybe it is her eyes which suddenly stare forward as if she has gone blind. Her body freezes like a statue, and even though she does not talk, I know something is terribly wrong, that my whole world is shaking at its very foundation.

Often I rest with Rebekah at night and encourage her to sleep. I pull her close and glance across at her face which is profiled in the room's glow. Her eyes are open. Her soft hair falls on my arm.

September 11, 1987

Friday. On Monday I undergo surgery. Deciding to have this operation has been difficult, but Gordon and I feel it is the only way to long-term health and peace of mind. I am past the point of terror, and there is a deep comfort somewhere beneath my anxiety.

I suppose I am confronting my mortality. Death seems directly in front of me. Yet I step into the sunlight surrounding my house into the field, thistles, and pampas grass, and I walk. Life, too, is in front of me.

Just now I wish I could drive Route 7, a secluded road running northbound from Morgantown into Pennsylvania. Once I drove that precipitous, winding route when I needed to sort thoughts. Autumn hay in pastures, stone walls and hedges bordering fields, new growth of the rhododendron that many had predicted would die after the winter's chill. A sign: "Clinton No. 7 Mine." There was no shaft or tipple in view, no evidence of men moving in the shadows below. I remember a barn filled with straw, a white house where a woman plays with a child on a wooden porch. Why can't I feel now the way I felt then?

September 13, 1987

Today I enter the hospital. But first I am at church, at sacrament meeting. It does help to be here, although it is difficult to engender and sustain a sense of spirituality. While it might be easier to well up with positive thinking, or with despair, or to listen to my emotions, I must attend to spiritual feelings. The peaceful atmosphere, the familiar songs, and sounds of children coalesce. I see the black nest that hangs on a window ledge of our home and hear the birds. But I can't sustain this energy. I can't give up my fear. A woman speaks to the congregation. She smiles. Gordon jots something on a small pad of paper, and Rebekah presses her shoulder into my arm.

September 24, 1987

It has been almost two weeks since my operation. The part I dread most about surgery is the recovery room, the anesthesia, that feeling of fading in and fading out, of trying to push back into being. "Breathe, Elizabeth," a nurse said loudly, "Breathe!"

I was cold. My friend Phyllis Updike, who was there, said my teeth chattered until the nurses covered me with foil. Phyllis, herself a nurse, sat on my right side, Gordon on my left. Leaning above me, their faces appeared and disappeared.

I needed to know something. I struggled to find thought, to find words. Finally the words came:

"What happened with the freeze-section?"

"The surgery went just fine," Gordon said softly.

Gathering my thoughts again I asked, "What happened with the freeze-section?"

"I think you better tell her," Phyllis said.

"It was positive wasn't it?" I asked.

"Yes."

Strange—in learning that I relaxed and fell back into the dark.

Gordon was waiting in the University Hospital Administrator's office, visiting with the Medical School Dean. Three doctors in green walked into the room: a plastic surgeon, a cancer surgeon, and an internist.

Doctor Ketch, the plastic surgeon, said, "We've got a problem. This thing is cancerous. We need to know what you want us to do."

Gordon told me that he cried out. In my mind I hear that quick, pained response, almost like a high-pitched laugh. Maybe the cry came when the doctors confirmed the cancer, or maybe it was after they left, and I can't recall how I know of it, but the sound haunts me.

I am experiencing much discomfort and pain. The surgery was extensive, a shock to my body. My head is still fogged. It is hard to think, hard to write, hard to remember what it was like to walk in the field by our home.

September 25, 1987

We all have colds. We went to bed early, but I awoke in the middle of the night and could not get back to sleep. This happens a lot. I sleep for a while, then bolt awake. My skin becomes hot, and my veins throb. My heart seems to beat irregularly. I am afraid to close my eyes. The association is of death. When one dies, does the room just go dark? Do we slip from a blue room into one that is black?

The pain is less than in the hospital where the days following surgery were filled with endless discomfort. Dr. Ketch said, "You're going to hurt," and he was right. When the morphine wore off, a deep tightness like the teeth of a trap gripped my chest. It's still hard to move. I lie on my side, supported by pillows. One holds my knees off of the mattress, and another keeps my arm away from my incisions. The pressure against my rib cage is tremendous, as though one side of my body were being pulled through the other.

September 26, 1987

Rebekah is cheerful this morning. Her hair is newly permed. Clearly she is taking more interest in her appearance than she did six months ago. She will be twelve soon and seems to be sweeping through adolescence. I am growing stronger. This morning I walked forty minutes in the field without tiring. It seems that the more I am able to walk, the more I heal. Walking is one way that I connect with life. When I walk, I feel myself moving through the world, traveling a course of time, space, and consciousness. I study nature, encounter people, smell a chrysanthemum. My minds goes back to the flowerbeds that Jack Miller and I passed on our walk to second grade, bright orange and yellow flowers dusted by gold moths. A bike moves toward me. Then a couple, walking three dogs, approaches from behind. The dogs run in circles through the field, and I drop behind to let them move a comfortable distance away. Now my attention shifts to the huge, pink rock formations of the Flatiron Mountains. It is amazing to be alive, to feel my hamstring muscles stretch, touch leaves and branches, love a husband, talk to my own child, actually believe, really believe that there is a God.

I know a woman who paints in her journal. It helps her to see, to better comprehend her world: delicate trees, bark, paint that is peeling, and soft laughter. Walking is my way of painting in a journal, so to speak, of seeing.

September 27, 1987

Today I am writing out some new life goals, trying to think hopefully about the future. I have had a hard time thinking forward in time without driving into a mound of rough stone waiting to be carved into tombstones. Often, I hear music, see someone standing at a pulpit, see my face in a coffin. My make-up is thick and orange. The hair is wrong, a 1950s mass of poufs. My dress has lace around the collar, such as women often wear in a Mormon temple. Can't I wear a white blazer with nice shoulder pads and a soft, wool crepe skirt that reaches to my ankles? I am haunted by the coffin closing on my face, the light becoming a line, and then everything black.

But there is also a new restlessness within me, an urge to fly like a gull perched on a bleached log who then lifts and glides over breaking water.

My mother has been with us since the surgery. I hear her and Rebekah return from church. Rebekah complains that it was too long.

She missed church last week and now remarks, "I guess I haven't built up my immune system for long meetings." Rebekah and Mother love to bake, and tonight they are going to make shortbread. For a few minutes, I will watch them work. Rebekah's voice rises and falls with excitement. Cupboards open, close. Utensils clink. Mother presses a rolling pin, and flat yellow dough comes out one side.

September 30, 1987

The red scars and stiff flesh around my surgery are modifying who I am. Is this what Hemingway meant when he said, ". . . the cold rains kept on and killed the spring . . ."? I am starting to realize that I have breast cancer. Will I die like my friend Nancy? One day I heard she had breast cancer. In three weeks she was dead. It didn't seem so bad for her. She wanted only to die at home and in her husband's arms. She got those wishes. Her friends came to see her. "I should have died before I lived," she told them in those final moments.

Looking at my body, I know that it's changed, but I can't bear thinking about the consequence or to write about it in my journal. Right now, sexuality seems a small matter compared to the larger desperation that I feel. I don't know how to put my life together again. I don't want to bog down in self-pity. But where do I begin? Perhaps I can change, grow, reach to a deeper self. If I don't learn and grow from my experience, then I am left only with a disaster. I fear drifting back into an old oblivion where life is taken for granted and routine removes you from much of the vividness of nature. For now I procrastinate answering mail or working and give myself permission to do nothing for a while except read, write poetry, and go for long walks.

October 2, 1987

I can't believe that on top of my recent breast cancer surgery that I may have ruptured a disk in my back. When I had my hair done yesterday, my back began to hurt. Then this morning at my physical therapy appointment, my leg started to stiffen. The therapist lifted my left limb and then called in a physician who said the back symptoms do not look good.

The therapist is teaching me exercises that should return the mobility to my arms which was diminished by my cancer operation. I have a lot of stiffness along the underside of my arms and find it hard to rotate them into a straight, vertical position. One exercise I do in bed: I hold soup cans in each hand and reach them over my head and as far toward the headboard as possible. Because of my back problem, I must stay flat in bed today and tomorrow, so I will have plenty of time for soup-can calisthenics.

I am in bed now, and Rebekah just ran in to deliver my noon time meal and to tell me about her plans for shopping with her dad. Her voice rises as she talks about where they will go. For several hours, she will have his undivided attention, time that will help reassure her that someone is still there to take care of her. Her lips form a thin crescent as she positions small plates filled with green lettuce, carrot sticks, an apple, and a delicate blue teacup offering the aroma of mint tea.

October 3, 1987

Today Mother returned to Salt Lake. She has been with us since the surgery, for almost two-and-a-half weeks, and has been enormously helpful and generous with her time. It seems we drew closer because of my health problems. One night, when I cried after learning I would have to undergo chemotherapy, she put her arm around my shoulders and held me in a very comforting way. Mother's life has not been easy. At only thirty-three she was left a widow. Often I am by myself with Rebekah, so have some sense of the burdens of a single parent. When I think of Mother, I think of endless striving, being tired, getting the children to school, her going back to teaching school, then having extreme pain in her limbs, so that she could only sit on the edge of the bed in the morning, fold over her knees, and cry. She had to worry about finances, about having enough money to keep a family of three going. There was no compensation from the company that manufactured the plane that killed my father, and there was nothing to speak of in the way of insurance. She went to work as a secretary at the University of Utah, and at night came home and cooked and cleaned. She was appointed to the Primary General Board, a significant leadership position in our church, which meant she had to write books for children, speak at conferences, go to meetings at five in the morning. Yet she did have a caring family and parents, and that is what saved us, what gave her rest. When my father died, her parents, brothers, and sisters were there for us.

God has his own way. My grandparents knew. My mother knew. Mother always has had God. Each day, her heart fills with faith. Now I wish my belief could be that bright and pure.

October 4, 1987

Sunday. Gordon is in Washington at a conference. I was awake all last night. Every time I dropped off to sleep I dreamt of death and dying. In one dream, Rebekah and I were in an airplane that was about to crash. It went into a nose dive and could not pull out. Somehow we became observers and watched the plane slowly descend, although we did not witness any impact. Perhaps my father's death is in this. I often think what it must have been like for him in that cockpit the moment before his plane was demolished and he died. That, I keep thinking, was the type of moment when you surrender to God and know you are in His hands. Something in me imagines that God replaces terror with peace and that the space between mortality and immortality becomes very thin. Maybe His comfort holds you while you cross that short distance. There was another strange dream. It had something to do with placing a box on a railroad track. I think of the apparition in Tolstoy's *Anna Karenina* where, in a train yard, an old man raises a lantern as if to show death as a light that illuminates the way of life. In my dream, I think the box on the track symbolizes death.

Between dreams I was awake. I watched the sky change from night to day and the Flatiron rocks become visible. In recent weeks I have had little close human contact, or so it feels. My bedroom is not a place other people want to visit. But I don't blame them for staying away, and they don't even know that they do. It is not an inviting place even for Gordon and Rebekah: no cozy fire, no food, no television. Only a person whom, in one sense, they have lost.

October 5, 1987

The pain in my back is not dissipating and seems to be crowding my thoughts about breast cancer. I desperately want to think through what breast cancer means and figure how to get beyond nightmares like last night's: In my dream I could feel terrible pain near the spot of my cancer, a sharp burning that would fire to an unbearable level, and then fade. In agony I searched for the cause, finally noticing an incision which opened to reveal a small animal gnawing at my flesh.

October 8, 1987

My first chemotherapy treatment is tomorrow. My oncologist, Dr. Robinson, wants me to have six treatments because tests suggest that I have an aggressive form of cancer. Since I was persistent with self-examination, my cancer was caught early, when the tumor was small. All twenty-six nodes were removed and bore no evidence of metastasis, meaning that I have "stage one" cancer and a good chance at full recovery. Nevertheless, breast cancer is often more aggressive in younger women than for those who have passed menopause, so, generally, someone my age should be given adjuvent chemotherapy as an extra protection.

Gordon knows I am nervous, but he cannot comprehend how afraid I am about tomorrow, despite Dr. Robinson's assurance that most women tolerate treatment well. Cancer therapy is often described as "painful" but what does "painful" mean: pain around the tumor, in the limbs or stomach because of the nausea? All today, I imagine myself vomiting, eyes sunken, back hunched, my whole body thrown into jarring spasms.

October 9, 1987

My chemotherapy treatment today was actually quite easy, once I passed my initial fright. Gordon drove me to the Health Sciences Center in Denver, and I could tell by his silent manner that he shared my apprehension. When I walked into the waiting room, Linda, an oncology nurse, handed me a beautiful bouquet of white flowers that my friend Jeannie Fuller had sent. About five years ago, Jeannie had undergone breast cancer surgery and chemotherapy. Somehow the flowers with their yellow stamens and pale purple centers quieted my fears.

The treatment room was so cold that my veins would not dilate. Linda tried warming my arm with a hot pad, but the veins remained tight and thin. After several insertions of an I.V. needle, a line of blood started to fill the plastic tube connected to my arm. Then she started to inject the drugs—Cytoxan, Methotrexate, 5 FU—slowly pushing the yellow liquid from the syringe. While I lay on the examination table, Dr. Robinson and Gordon stood nearby—talking with each other, but also with Linda and me. The whole process took about fifteen minutes, and the only discomfort was a bit of itching that curiously followed one of the three injections. For a few minutes on the return trip to Boulder, I fell asleep, a result of the anti-nausea medication. Gordon just dropped me off at home and has returned to work. Right now I am feeling a little tired, my back is hurting terribly, and I can barely walk, so I will try working in bed until Rebekah comes home from school. Luckily, this looks like a night free of university work for me, although Gordon won't have time for dinner before his evening function. I think about how comforting it was to be with him today for a few hours, even just driving together to something we both feared.

October 10, 1987

I am becoming accustomed to living on a bed. The bedroom has become an office with books and writing materials all within arm's reach. Dictating equipment is close by, and a couple of law review articles that I wrote on legal ethics are scattered on the bed covers. They were accepted for publication more than a year ago. Of course it has to be this week that I receive the galley proofs and the publisher's requests to return them in a matter of days. I still cannot focus my eyes—or my thoughts—very well, let alone remember what I wrote eighteen months ago. So I decide to hire an editor to review the manuscripts and trust any corrections to her and to my assistant, Maggie. But first I am trying to make some sense out of these papers, struggling to follow my own analysis. The mind is not conditioned to function when the body is prone. The signal is to go to sleep, and I keep doing so.

A stack of get-well cards is growing. Besides working on the manuscripts, I try to write notes of thanks. Because my cancer was announced in the Colorado newspapers, I have received hundreds of cards from people I do not know. Some are lengthy letters, some are personal stories of like experiences. The thoughts and prayers of people are uplifting, voices that sustain my sense of presence at a time of frail courage. Consoling words flow through that central spirit vein that unites us all, that nerve of understanding that lights one's love and decreases dread.

Phyllis has been close to me since my surgery. During this past month, our friendship has been an easy flowering. She has been steady, and I have become open to her faithful care. Today she drove from Denver for a visit. We looked from the window and saw orange and yellow strands among green, and lush trees that reach all the way to the mountains.

Tonight Rebekah is baking. Baking has been her favorite activity for the past several months. She especially likes to make things that are lemon. I call them "lemon-everythings"—petit fours, meringue pie, cake, tea cookies.

October 13, 1987

Today I was examined by a neurologist who says I have a herniated disk and that I must go to bed. An intense pain radiates down my entire leg, focusing in my upper thigh. Rarely can I find a comfortable position during the day or night, so it's hard to work or sleep. Last evening I cried because I was so discouraged and fearful of undergoing another surgery, one of a different kind. Sometimes I wonder if my breast cancer has created this annoying problem.

Now on top of my new back problem, reporters want to talk with me about the cancer surgery. Someone even wanted to do an interview while I was still in the hospital. But I don't know how I feel about an interview right now. Will I lose control of my emotions? Nancy Reagan has just had breast cancer surgery, and because media interest has grown on the subject, I probably will consent to one interview with the local newspaper, hoping what I might say will prompt women to see their doctors and have a mammogram.

October 17, 1987

Saturday. I am still in bed because of this ruptured disk. I want to write in my journal about my breast cancer but find it too awkward. I can only lie flat on my back or on my sides, and it is almost impossible to coordinate pen and paper. My back has improved, but not a great deal. Because two of my nerves are impaired by the herniation, I have lost some reflexes.

I have been alone a lot lately. Gordon is often away fulfilling his duties as a university president, and Rebekah is in school a good part of the day. Being immobile and alone is hard. There is so much silence. It surrounds me. At first it feels warm and safe. Then it quietly turns cold, an empty sameness. I try to shake off the blankness, to feel thought and energy, but my mind is taken by the idleness, by the loneliness. I simply move from hour to hour, silence to silence, until someone comes and I am alive again.

October 21, 1987

I have returned to the hospital for an evaluation of my back problem. Unfortunately, I am not making significant progress and now need to seriously consider back surgery. Here in the hospital, unable to write, I dictate a journal entry into a tape recorder.

Rebekah and I had a bedtime telephone conversation. We did not talk long because she was late getting to bed. Since coming to the hospital, I have tried to communicate with her several times each day: At the least, we visit when she is just returning from school and before bed. Tonight we talked about her Halloween costume. This year, she is going to be a rabbit jumping out of a hat, although she considered being a cancan girl, university graduate, hospital patient, the Statue of Liberty, Christmas tree, or playing card. Nothing scary. At night we usually sing a song and talk about the day's events. This evening it was "The Moon and the Stars," a little tune I composed for her when she was small.

Our conversation was late today because Rebekah had to wash her hair and make a gift for the Curator of the Giza Pyramids and the Egyptian Minister of Antiquities. Gordon and I were to host a dinner in their honor at our home, but Rebekah will take my place. She seems excited. She made a banner welcoming them to Boulder and also a card and watercolor of a mask.

I spent the day with more dictation and notes of thanks. I tried reading Henry James' *Portrait of a Lady*, without much success, because I could not suspend the book over my head long enough. This morning, a nurse helped me wash my hair, which was a major undertaking as I had to remain flat in bed and position my head in a flat pan that drained the water into a plastic wastebasket. Two or three times a day I break into tears of frustration. I can't believe I am back in the hospital living with reminders of the breast cancer surgery: the faint blue glow of the nightlight; morning blood tests; a black, rubber sleeve tightened around my upper arm; and the monotone voice of the paging operator.

Why can't I be like the people who pass in and out of my room? The young medical students look so strong and healthy that I can almost see through their skin to pink, clean muscles and organs.

October 22, 1987

Last night was terrifying for me. The oncology nurse stopped by to check on me even though I am in the hospital for back problems. She had my breast cancer chart, and I asked if she would mind reviewing the pathology findings. When the doctors had first gone over them with me five weeks ago following surgery, I was still foggy from the anesthetic and did not exactly hear what they said. What the nurse now read seemed much worse than I originally recalled. The report describes the cancer as "invasive inter-ductile cancer," indicating that it had started to merge with the surrounding tissue in the mammary duct, although there was no evidence that it had penetrated the blood vessels. To me this sounded very serious, although the cancer was still marked as "stage one." I had thought the doctors said the cancer was contained or encapsulated, but now it sounded as though it was not and that it was starting to spread.

When the nurse left, I started to cry. I tried calling Gordon, but he was attending some university function. Suddenly I felt desperately alone in that dark hospital room. The halls glowed a faint blue, and in the next room a respirator exhaled and sucked with a scraping sound. Images of death crept closer and closer. My funeral. The songs. Flowers. The casket. My father lying in his coffin.

I was so upset that finally the night nurse called Dr. Byyny at home. It was close to ten in the evening. Patiently he listened to my review of the report. We talked for a long period, then he phoned the other physicians. That same night he called me to relate his conversations and to correct my misunderstandings. For the next day, he arranged a conference of all health care providers associated with my health problems, so that I could ask questions, be reassured, and understand the information I had been given. It was a very time-consuming, caring effort on his part.

November 5, 1987

There is an empty space in my journal. About two weeks ago my badly-ruptured disk was removed from my back. The doctors said the rupture was serious, and that I might as well have the surgery. Surprisingly, the operation was easy. I experienced no pain and, by the first evening, was making cheerful calls home. The next day I walked down the hospital corridors, feeling the weight of my body press into my calves and ankles. It was unbelievably good to feel gravity pull me into the soles of my feet.

The surgery was timed between chemotherapy treatments. I was given my second chemotherapy treatment while in the hospital. It took four tries and about fifteen minutes for them to get the needle into a vein. By the time the tubes were in place, I was almost in shock. Five days after back surgery, I returned home, only to discover that we were entertaining three hundred guests that evening. When the party started, I went to my bedroom where I could lie down and visit with Rebekah. We listened to the voices fill the room below and once in awhile peeked out of the window to watch shadows move behind the living room blinds. A couple of times Gordon ran upstairs to see how I was doing, and every few minutes someone else would pop into the room—a gift-bearing guest, a caterer offering refreshments, a staff member asking about a misplaced tray. By the end of the evening, I was exhausted, but also felt reconnected to my family and this house.

❧ *Echoes from the Field*

November 8, 1987

I have the doctor's permission to start walking in the field. As I follow the narrow dirt path, I realize that I have missed a whole season. When I first entered the hospital in mid-September, the trees were in full leaf: aspen and birch branches were heavy with foliage, so leaves touched leaves, layers touched layers. Now only a few dry, yellow flakes are strung along thin boughs, the air is not that of fall, but of approaching winter. The sky is cold, full of wind. All around there are shadows, and the warm air is gone.

November 10, 1987

Finally I am starting to sleep a little better even though the nightmares are persisting. At least I am not waking every few hours with the intense bands of pressure across my chest from the cancer surgery or sharp leg pains resulting from a ruptured disk. Also, Gordon must be getting more rest at night because he no longer turns over or asks, "Are you OK?" every time I move my legs or strain to see the glowing hands of the clock on the night stand. Thankfully, my physical discomfort seems to be on the decline. The psychological healing, however, will be a slower process. But that is all right, I will need time to understand this breast cancer and the physical, emotional, and spiritual transformation it is bringing. It's funny how I feel that I have been waiting for this time, how when Gordon answered "yes" to my question in the recovery room about the freeze section that I knew the moment had come for a new life quest. Even in that dreamless stupor I felt a spark of exhilaration, perhaps something like soldiers feel when they yell a battle cry.

November 11, 1987

Today I drove to Denver for a photo session. I am giving Gordon a portrait for Christmas. While I tell myself it will be nice for his office, I also know it's for in case I die, so he will have a recent photograph of me. It was not an easy trip because I had to drive a long distance and then sit in an uncomfortable position for a half an hour, but I finally made it through. Now I am looking forward to bed. This evening Rebekah played with Eva, a friend from Sweden who is attending Burbank Junior High this year. Earlier, the three of us stopped by Safeway to buy a magazine. It was a treat to be able to go to a supermarket after so long an absence. Walking up and down the aisles or passing the frozen foods, I enjoyed the clinking of grocery carts and frigid air touching my skin.

November 16, 1987

Since July, we have been living in the new University of Colorado president's home, but some final decorating decisions remain. Because of my illness and university obligations that just won't wait, I have not been able to devote much time or energy to getting the house in order.

Today I surveyed the university's art collection to see if there might be some pieces we could exhibit in the residence. Then I took a brief walk across campus. Yesterday, it snowed and the campus is especially beautiful. For several minutes, I rested on a small stone bench and ran my hand along a tree trunk, then through a dry clump of red leaves. Each texture registered inside me. When the sun made yellow lines on snow-covered branches, I knew that I would remember these simple, indelible patterns.

November 17, 1987

This morning I am spending some time in my law school office. Although I am not employed by the law school, the university gave me a small office here because the university residence is too busy a place for doing serious work—one day when I was home in bed I counted over one hundred incoming telephone calls. This is a quiet place where I come to catch up on paperwork, make telephone calls, and write. It feels good to be here and return to the life I left two months ago.

Before going in, I stayed in the car several minutes. First I said my morning prayer, and then lowered the windows just to enjoy the sights, sounds, and smells of nature: sun on snow, birds fighting at a window feeder, law students conversing, pink patterns in the flagstone of the buildings, colors in a piece of gravel. These seem a good entry point for re-experiencing the world, a way of restoring some coherence to the scattered pieces of my life.

November 23, 1987

It does not seem a month and a half since my breast cancer surgery and three weeks since my back surgery. I feel so good that sometimes I forget about the operations, but then I lift or bend, and a sharp pain reminds me. Today I attended church yet stayed for only one hour because my back was tired. We sat by a woman wearing strong perfume which caused Rebekah to immediately become congested, making her miserable throughout the meeting. Rebekah has a lot of nervous energy, and it is hard for her to sit through our Sunday service under the best of circumstances. It was difficult to have any spiritual feelings sitting next to a wheezing, complaining child. Yet I sympathized with her.

Rebekah's friend, Lisa Connely, is staying with us while her parents are in Tucson, Arizona. This evening, the girls baked a lemon cake to take to a school party the next day, but Rebekah accidentally dropped it. Slowly it slid off the tray and splatted on the floor. Her pained eyes caught mine, and for a moment I remembered how fragile children are. Quickly, I promised to make a replacement, and the girls moved on to baking lemon meringue pie—crust and all. Today a boy came to the house to visit Rebekah and Lisa. They played in the snow and generally seemed to have a good time, but as soon as he left, they pronounced him a "real dip."

For church today, Rebekah wore her yellow sweater and skirt purchased this summer in London. I am noticing that she is now interested in clothing. This season her favorite items are a "Hard Rock Cafe" T-shirt and a yellow, felt hat covered with pins that she collected on our family trips. Until this year, Rebekah would wear nothing but pastel sweat suits. Now they hang in the closet like wilting petals, their sweet order shaken by jeans and black denim. Somehow, she seems to be stepping away from me, moving to a new kind of liberty. There is a lightness kindling within her. I lie next to her at night. Two wide eyes face me on the pillow, and even in silence I sense her motion.

November 24, 1987

Today, I am reviewing our commitments for holiday entertaining. It will be full, as it always is, with six or seven functions at the residence of one kind or another: afternoon and evening receptions, dinner parties, luncheons. Our home social schedule was reduced some in the months following my surgery, so that I could simply recover and

Gordon could help out a little more. Now we are moving back into our normal university routines, although I wish we could delay a little while longer. Usually, I feel tired, especially in the evening, and by the time I get to bed I am close to exhaustion. But more than needing sleep, I want some quiet space in the day to let ordinary moments linger, to put a golden frame around each step I take in the field, each word of my quiet conversations with Gordon, each note of Rebekah's morning songs.

November 26, 1987

I had my third chemotherapy treatment. This time, I did not vomit as I did after the second treatment. I am taking a different anti-nausea medication and avoiding rich foods—my downfall last time. I will stick with Cream of Rice, Popsicles, and scraped apples.

Grandma Cannon believed in scraped apples. I can envision her cutting them into quarters and gently scraping small mounds of pulp from each section. She sits by me, patiently paring the fruit until there is a soft morsel of magic foam that makes me well. It takes a long time to eat an apple this way. But it makes my skin warm. Don't ask me how. Then she tells me stories, about Hans Brinker or about "Seven Dancing Princesses," and I can see to that time, to ice on the canal, the trees filled with glittering sapphires. A dim light follows her to the pantry where she opens glass cupboard doors. A pattern of light falls on them. On the shelves are china plates, cool and smooth, the texture of the inside of a sea shell. She stands over me, her reflection in the window.

November 27, 1987

We are spending part of Thanksgiving weekend in Breckenridge, Colorado, at our mountain home—our very necessary refuge from our demanding public lives. The university residence is like an office building open to workers. I sometimes feel that a hierarchy of watchers has come to observe our every move there. On autumn days, I long for a place to have mint tea and sit alone by a fire. In the morning, I travel to my small windowless office in the law school. Its "windows" are several art pieces and art books. A life-size Fauvist sculpture broods in a corner, and three clay masks molded by Rebekah stare at me across the desk. Still, there are times when I would rather be home and let the afternoon sun fall on my face while Rebekah sits nearby watching cartoons.

It is easier for Gordon. He is naturally outgoing and social, and thrives in a public world. His idea of a good time, I tell friends, is a reception for four hundred people. Gordon is as invigorated by public contact as I am by geese in an approaching storm. You can see him reach out into the crowd. You can feel his exuberance.

November 29, 1987

Most of Thanksgiving Day, we just relaxed in the beautiful mountain surroundings. Snow fell on the trees and pond. While still awake long after Gordon and Rebekah had gone to sleep, I thought about dying and watched white branches turn whiter. A thin haze fell into the woods.

Several times today I stepped onto the front deck just to be there and to be alive. I curled my fingers around some pine needles. They felt smooth and polished as I pulled my hand along the branch and off the end. I took a breath of smoke that was coming down the roof from the fireplace.

On Friday, we outfitted Rebekah for skiing. This is a challenge because she is difficult to please. Every other store in Breckenridge is a ski shop, and we must have gone to half of them. Her primary concern was color. Finding ski clothing in pastel hues which fit her was no small task. A "small" in a woman's jacket fits, but the matching pants fall off of her hips. Eventually, she triumphed with white, lavender, and peach. We celebrated our success with lunch at "Tillies" (great onion rings) and with the purchase of a stuffed flamingo for Rebekah's up-coming "fifties" birthday party.

On Friday we returned home to attend the Saturday University of Colorado/Nebraska football game. It was a sunny, socially successful day, even though the team did not win. Gordon and I host brunches for several hundred people prior to each football game, and today our guests were especially kind to me, seeing me back on my feet. Tears welled in my eyes several times—my emotions still unpredictable in public.

December 1, 1987

I reported to my job at the Center for Health Ethics and Policy at the University of Colorado in Denver. This is the first full day I have worked since my surgery in October. The Center is a new university entity that will conduct research and direct programs focusing on bioethical and health policy problems. For almost a year I have been involved in planning the Center and securing its funding. For the time being, I am employed as a Senior Research Associate with responsibilities for program development, teaching, and administration. I also do research which currently focuses on pressing social problems that to-day are euphemized as "ethical dilemmas," particularly in the fields of law and medicine.

Because I had to leave the house early this morning I did not do my aerobic walking, journal writing, or Scripture reading—a relaxing and rejuvenating routine I began during my illness. I need to find ways to keep these things in my daily schedule. Assuredly, they set the tone for the day, and when I fail to follow this pattern I feel unsettled. But even so, I have a sense of living "in the moment" while working in the Center's offices which are on the fifth floor of a new building. My large window overlooks the city's skyline: orange-red forms, some in shadows, some in morning light, rise into a blue sky. The sun is high, and bland sides of featureless buildings are in focus. Below, two men in T-shirts lean against the wall of a dark cafe, lighting cigarettes while cars curve around the corner onto Larimer Street then accelerate and scatter.

December 2, 1987

Last night, at our home in Boulder, I could not sleep, so I stepped onto the bedroom deck to see the moon. It was a soft alabaster like the bisque face of a doll a friend of my mother's gave me when I was five. The air was still and cold. But high above, wind swept the clouds into curls. I stood looking until the picture had blown away. Moving into the warm bedroom, images of Grandpa and Grandma Cannon and also my father, loved ones who have passed away, filled my thoughts. I wondered if they are experiencing anything at all.

The doctor said not to fight the sleeplessness and, instead, use it as time to work through the past months. I have arranged a little table in the guest room where I sit after Gordon and Rebekah are asleep. On the table are a scented candle, notebook, and pencil—this is where I go to think, write, and consider obscure feelings.

December 5, 1987

New York City. We're on our annual Christmas trip, a holiday tradition we began in West Virginia from where we could fly to New York in a few hours. We enjoy the Christmas season in New York City so much that we spend four or five days here each December. In many respects, we are typical vacationers, shopping, visiting museums, and going to Broadway productions. But even to Rebekah the city has become familiar, so the tourist attractions are no longer so much on our route. This is my first "outing" since my surgeries, and it seems unbelievably wonderful to actually be taking a trip with Rebekah and Gordon.

Yesterday we visited Sir Brian Urquart, former Deputy Secretary General of the United Nations. Our mission was to deliver a memento from when the University honored him this past year. He took us to lunch at the U.N. and then on a tour of the building. He was an immediate friend to Rebekah and let her stand behind the podium in the General Assembly room. As I stood watching her—there were only four of us in the hall—time seemed to freeze. My eyes followed along the dark blue walls that formed a wide arch so high that the ceiling's light fixtures were hardly visible. From a central aisle, empty desks made of smooth cherry curved out like ribs, reminding me of something Teilhard de Chardin said about "society as an organism." The room felt alive. That evening, the nightly news showed Soviet leader Mikhail Gorbachev at the same podium.

Rebekah is very inquisitive, and often she and Sir Brian would venture down some hall by themselves to examine tapestries or artifacts donated by various countries. They studied gold fabric from India, antique porcelain from China. Former U.N. Secretary, Kurt Waldheim, has been in the news lately in connection with his Nazi involvement, and at lunch we discussed Waldheim's failure to disclose his Nazi association. Mr. Urquart felt bitterly deceived by Waldheim, especially because he knew him personally. But the next moment we were laughing at his story of being knighted by Queen Elizabeth and how he stood in line like a ticket holder waiting for the honor.

December 6, 1987

The stores in New York are decorated for the holidays, many with artificial pine boughs and white lights winding around enormous pillars. Some of the trimmings are about the same as when Gordon and I lived here twenty years ago. There is a particular scent in the stores this time each year, a blending of perfume, damp clothing, and chocolate.

Today I spent a lot of time sitting in Bloomingdale's and Macy's juniors departments, more time than I would have liked. I know that it is exciting for a young girl to browse through rows of clothing, so I try to give her a few chances to do so. Rebekah quickly moved back and forth between the dressing room and racks of colorful shirts. Leaning against a low counter, I began seeing horrifying images of hospitals and funerals. I'm amazed at how quickly cancer has staked out a wide territory in my ordinary thoughts and daydreams.

December 7, 1987

I have several books of poetry in my office. Today, back in Boulder, I was flipping through a collection of poems by W. H. Auden and caught the title, "Miss Gee." It was a poem about cancer and, with my name on it, uncomfortably ironic. It is written like a nursery rhyme, I thought, perhaps to establish contrast between the telling of the story and its real horror. The narrator speaks in a child's taunting voice, like that heard on a playground when children tease each other. Miss Gee has cancer and soon finds herself on an operating table, helpless as a child and surrounded by laughing boys who playfully regard her advanced sarcoma. Miss Gee dies, and they suspend her cadaver from the ceiling.

December 9, 1987

This morning I drove to Denver for a chest X-ray, blood test, and a visit with Dr. Byyny, my internist, about scheduling frequent examinations, so that I might be reassured about the progress of my health. I still have two small breast lumps that appeared after surgery which must be monitored. Next, I saw the two surgeons who operated on me for cancer. While they were not concerned about these problem areas, I remember the same "unconcern" preceded my last surgery. The fact is that there has been no time in the last twenty years when my doctors have not been watching something that could be breast cancer. Often I think about other women like myself, how breast cancer inhabits their lives, how it seems to be a net thrown over their most intimate thoughts, fears, and dreams. It is a web so persistent and present that its grip becomes familiar, a given part of daily existence.

Last night I dreamed about a Christmas tree covered with decorations representing death. I don't precisely remember what they looked like. I just recall ghoulish ornaments hanging from thin, silver threads, chiseled jewels that glowed vaguely as light. Lying there, stretched out on sheets damp with perspiration, I looked out the window at a night that opened onto the field. Despite these difficult times, I do feel that I am improving.

December 11, 1987

Tonight is Rebekah's twelfth birthday party, and it was wonderful to see her happy and free from the stress of the past months. Having chosen a "fifties" theme for the celebration, she asked the ten friends she invited to the party to wear costumes. Katie Wise had a "pageboy" wig and jeweled spectacles turned up at the corners. Most of the girls wore full, mid-calf skirts and bobby socks, although a few dressed in "pedal pushers." Rebekah was intent on finding just the right outfit. At a used clothing store downtown, "Golden Oldies," she purchased a turquoise skirt with raised embroidered people and animals playing on a grassy field. A bolero-style sweater was bordered with a two-inch trim of white beads and sequins, reminding me of one that I had at her age. I wore it with a wide, red, elastic belt that I cinched tightly around my waist to make me look as though I had hips. I also remember wearing thick white socks and oxfords to the Sixth Avenue drugstore where my best friend, Jeannie Stevens, and I would sit at the counter on red stools and order lime-phosphates served in tall, slender glasses. We made our drinks last for hours. When we were through, we might spend an entire afternoon looking at the latest shades of nail polish and lipstick. From behind the counter, the sales clerk would hand us miniature sample tubes that entertained us for hours.

I was twelve the summer that my older cousin, Lou Jean Willis, and I decided that our lipstick should be the lightest color possible. We bought stick tubes of make-up used to cover blemishes and smeared it on our lips. Once we were visiting our Grandpa Cannon in his downtown office when Woody, the elevator operator, told us that we looked terrible with white lips. He was sixteen, very handsome, and the target of a good deal of flirtation. Lou Jean and I were devastated.

Tonight Rebekah's birthday party began with hamburgers, french fries, onion rings, and shakes, followed by chocolate cake, ice cream, and presents. The cake was decorated with a pink convertible and palm tree.

Rebekah did not want to cut into the convertible but eventually had to slice off the rear wheels. Then the girls took turns "lip-synching" to "fifties" music. Some sang together, others went it alone. Finally, they had a hula hoop and a bubble-blowing contest. Now three of the girls are staying overnight. I am going to bed! Tonight was fun, which makes me think I am starting to become myself again.

December 14, 1987

An important life goal for me has become good health. This means more sleep, balanced meals, exercise, and eliminating stress. Finding more time for sleep is difficult because Gordon requires very little and always must be prodded to come to bed, which usually is about midnight. Then he gets up at 5:30 A.M. to exercise and get Rebekah off to school. For the past few months, I have been staying in bed until about 7:30 A.M., and sometimes later. Probably I still tire more easily than before my surgeries because I do not sleep soundly.

I continue to walk almost two miles a day. When the weather is good, I walk in the field behind our home. First I go west, in the direction of the mountains, then north along the bike path. I return to the house, tracing my steps, and then take the same route one more time. Since the weather has been cold, I have been using the walking machine we keep in our upstairs loft. I cannot go much of a distance on the treadmill because I get bored. But also I prefer to walk outside because my awareness shifts to the new levels I have experienced in recent months. My favorite time is dusk when I can smell the damp grass, apple trees, and pines. When the air is still, the fragrances don't blend but instead hold together. Passing through these zones of sweet oxygen, I think I smell their feathered edges.

December 17, 1987

In a few days I will have the fourth of six chemotherapy treatments. This morning another handful of hair came out in the shower. Even

Rebekah said she can tell my hair is thinning because my part has widened into a clear line of pink skin. And yet, Dr. Robinson indicated that most breast cancer patients who receive the drugs that I am getting do not need wigs and that more than thirty percent hair loss would be atypical. Before I began treatment he advised me to purchase an inexpensive wig, as an insurance policy in case I should lose large amounts of hair. Eventually, I contacted a few beauty parlor operators and ordered two wigs made of synthetic hair: One is about chin length and the other several inches longer. When they arrived, I tried them on but was horrified at how ridiculous I looked. There would be no question that I was wearing a hairpiece since they had the texture of doll hair and neither sat well on my head. I knew I could never wear these wigs.

I don't know why hair is so important to self-image but it is. One of the ways the Nazis tortured Jewish women was to shave their heads. My friend who lost her hair to chemotherapy said she never looked at herself without her wig. She always put it on first thing every morning, struggling without the use of a mirror to pull it into place.

December 21, 1987

The chemotherapy treatment was not so bad. Gordon drove me to Denver, as he has every month, even though it often means canceling important appointments. The anti-nausea medication that comes with the drugs causes immediate drowsiness, and clearly it would be unsafe for me to drive home alone. Although several friends have offered to chauffeur me, I want to be with Gordon. The fact is that it helps to have his support because I dread returning to the hospital where I had surgery and being in a room filled with cancer patients. The last time I was there, a young woman in her twenties had covered her head with a colorful bandanna. Someone told me that she is a medical student with a malignant brain tumor, a kind almost always fatal. She smiled and joked with doctors and people who passed through the waiting room.

Because I have small, deep veins that are hard to tap, I have come to hate the insertion of the I.V. My first treatments involved numerous passes into my hand and forearm before the needle would connect with the vein. Now the nurses no longer insert the needle, and Dr. Robinson positions it himself. He never misses. "He can find a blood vessel in a grapefruit," the nurses remark. I sometimes feel like a grapefruit. In about ten days, I will go to the University of Colorado Student Health Center in Boulder for a white cell count. Since chemotherapy destroys both cancer cells and cells that fight infection, the white cell count must be monitored and should return to normal levels before more chemotherapy is given. Between treatments, I have at least two blood tests, and sometimes three. By now it seems that the veins in my arms are beginning to give out: Scar tissue is forming at the site of frequent needle punctures, and there is always a bad bruise on the inside of one arm or the other.

December 23, 1987

It has been snowing hard all day, so I canceled a morning appointment to discuss a project for work that deals with medical malpractice. I did drive to the Health Sciences Center to have a new small lesion in my left breast examined. Although the doctors feel certain it is not cancer, sometimes I wonder if they are trained to tell you the best until the arrival of the worst.

For several hours, I have been home and just finished some Christmas wrapping. I notice that the house is unusually quiet—no telephone calls or deliveries—and then I remember that it is December twenty-third and the University is slowing down until New Year's. A few minutes ago, Gordon arrived. He seems relaxed, as if he is starting to shift to a state of mind which is free of worries about work. We're viewing a movie starring Mickey Rooney about Christmas in New York. While Rebekah stirs hot fudge, we watch and visit in the kitchen. Yesterday she made shortbread cookies and candies, and now we have a beautiful Christmas plate of goodies.

Several times today I just took in the world and the joy of living each single moment. Rebekah and I played Christmas carols on the piano, then we stood on the bedroom deck together and watched the snow as it fell.

December 26, 1987

Christmas has been busy, but alive in its celebrations. I had hoped to write in my journal more, but when I am not in my normal work-study rhythm I forget important patterns such as Scripture study, and even walking. I need to better maintain my regular morning sequence, because it does set a tone for the day.

I have been remembering a herd of elk I saw in Rocky Mountain National Park, how they stood in a clearing searching side by side in the dark for red, withered leaves. I think about my loved ones and then how the elk move through the wilderness from year to year, winter to spring, how they are born and die with each other, how day after day they hold together. There is grandeur in this world and in the natural bonds of life that almost escape expression. William Carlos Williams said:

> *save in a poem*
> *shall it go*
> *to suffer no diminution*
> *of its splendor*

Although we often spend Christmas alone, because most of our relatives live in Utah, we always feel a close spirit with them. And even if other family members are not with us, they occupy our thoughts. While arranging Santa's gifts, I think of Mother reading *The Big Green Umbrella*, or of the sweet aroma of Grandma Cannon's chokecherry jelly boiling and spitting on the stove. Little radish leaves pierce the tilled soil in Aunt Jean and Uncle Bertram's vegetable garden. I kneel on a hard stool and bend over the kitchen sink while Nana, my father's mother, pours a cold vinegar rinse from a Mason jar over my hair. I smell the wet wood from the irrigation well in Nana and Poppy's back yard, ride in my father's new green Cadillac, taste Grandma Cannon's caramels and lemon-custard ice cream, gather horse chestnut blossoms for paper May baskets. I think of lavender and gold irises Rebekah planted in the back yard, telephone calls from summer camp, hands clasped in family prayer, Gordon's forehead pressing my cheek, *Anne of Green Gables* at bedtime. I remember frozen lime pie and doll houses. Just before dusk on Christmas Eve, a beautiful snowfall began and continued through the night. We had a white, white Christmas, opened presents, ate breakfast, called grandparents. We prayed a little and told each other we were glad for this day.

December 29, 1987

Gordon, Rebekah, and I are in Miami attending the Orange Bowl, although initially I did not plan to go on this trip. Gordon is expected to attend every Orange Bowl, regardless of whether or not University of Colorado's team played, and last January he and Rebekah made the trip alone. Then I stayed home, so that they could have some time together; but this time I came with them, afraid to be away when I feel an almost desperate need to stay close to them.

When we arrived last night, Florida was cold and windy and we took refuge at a shopping mall across from the hotel. Rebekah was fond of Mrs. Grimble's Restaurant where they serve quiche, thick soups, and rich cheesecake. When Gordon and I lived in New York twenty years ago, "Mrs. Grimble's" cheesecake was a favorite treat. I even remember the first time I sampled it: Frank and Mary Anne Walwer had invited us to dinner at their Manhattan apartment. At that time, Frank was Associate Dean of the Columbia University Law School, and Gordon was working as his research assistant. Why I was so impressed with the menu, I have no idea. Maybe it was that law deans and faculty seemed larger than life, but I recall that Mary Anne served rice-filled grape leaves, mellow fillet mignon (carved at the table), golden Yorkshire pudding, and Mrs. Grimble's raspberry-swirl cheesecake. For years, I have tried to duplicate this dinner on special occasions.

With the temperature in Florida somewhat improved today, we are able to enjoy the beach. Rebekah and a friend play in the surf and gather shells while I watch them run up and down from my hotel window. Earlier in the morning, I accompanied Gordon to a brunch for the university held at an ocean-front mansion, one of the many Orange Bowl social events. Then later on he watched Rebekah, so that I could shop for bargains. While I did find some nice jackets, I spent most of the time looking for a store that sold wigs. For a month now, I have continued to lose hair to the point that I think I simply must purchase a hairpiece. It occurred to me that there might be a store in the vicinity of the shopping mall. After a few inquiries, I was directed to a shop that had a rather unassuming window display with several old mannequins adorned with long flowing or bouffant-style wigs. I told the salesperson that I was losing my hair and needed a wig, and that I would be in town only a day or two. At this I was greeted with great kindness and ushered into the salon area of the store. The proprietor, Regina, came to assist me. Immediately, I recognized her face in photographs that covered every inch of wall space, although she was at least twenty years older than the most recent picture. Obviously she had been a make-up artist for one of the major networks as she was shown standing next to any number of great motion picture stars of the nineteen fifties: Cary Grant, Greta Garbo, Doris Day, to name a few. She was also photographed with Harry Truman, Walter Cronkite, and Joe DiMaggio wearing the same beehive hairdo she has today. All her wigs are natural hair, which is what I needed. It would be expensive, but a nice human hair wig would not look artificial. After trying several styles, I finally chose a hairpiece that just covered the top of my head and left what natural hair remained to fall naturally. Regina matched my color exactly and agreed to rush the order. By the following day, I had my new hair and a restored sense of equilibrium.

January 6, 1988

Almost four months since surgery, and I believe I am starting to mend both physically and psychologically, although a thought of death still frequently passes through my view. I try to think positive by visualizing myself alive in five, ten, or twenty years: I ask what Rebekah's high school graduation will be like, how I will feel when we drive her to college the first time, what kinds of things I will do with my grandchildren, if I will be able to achieve the professional accomplishments that are my goal.

When I awake, I thank God for another twenty-four hours of life. Throughout the day, I reflect on the life and world I am experiencing: I feel the texture of my skin, press my cheek against a leaf, or stroke Rebekah's hair. I listen to her sing as she dresses. I notice the grinding and swaying of a bus ride, the sensation of a hot shower on my back, or the taste of chocolate melting in my mouth.

January 14, 1988

The past week has been filled with many demands. Rebekah will be having final examinations next week, and so much of my home time has been spent helping her prepare. Now I am working in Denver four days a week, putting in quite full days. Even though my job is not terribly stressful, I am tired when I return, probably because the chemotherapy treatments are sapping my physical energy.

I am still getting settled in my new office which I will have to share for a brief time. It has two desks and looks and feels junky: Brown boxes are stacked on top of one another, my clothes snag on Formica that protrudes from the bookcase, a fine dust covers everything and is on my hands and in my lungs.

Getting back into a professional routine is good therapy, however frustrating. This Ethics Center is the third I have helped start, and working on another helps me connect with the life I led before surgery. Yet, I do feel differently about being here, about having this career. Often I wonder where this path leads and how it fits with the rest of my life.

My immediate responsibilities at the Ethics Center are planning a staff retreat, editing the Center's newsletter, serving as a senior staff assistant to the director during the start-up phase, developing fund-raising strategies, preparing grant proposals, coordinating staff and policy review board meetings, serving as a liaison with other university departments, teaching, and conducting research. I requested that my appointment be only three-quarters time! Indeed my schedule needed to leave room for family and my responsibilities as a university president's spouse.

Although I must now drive between Boulder and Denver four times a week, I do not particularly mind the ride because it is my only quiet time during the day. Sometimes I listen to the _Book of Mormon_ on cassette tapes, other times I play recordings of books or listen to the news on public radio. Driving time is a chance for reflection, when I concentrate on the experience of living, and notice the fields of grazing cattle, the mountains in the distance, and the folds of gray clouds in the sky above the plains.

January 17, 1988

Last night Gordon spoke at the fiftieth anniversary of the Cortez Chamber of Commerce and did not get home until 1:30 A.M. He said he thought he shook every hand in the town. Knowing that he would be coming in late, I decided to sleep in the guest room. I was afraid if I slept in the master bedroom that I would awaken when he returned and then not be able to get back to sleep. When Gordon noticed I wasn't in bed, he deduced that I was with Rebekah and so set the security system which went off when I turned in my sleep. The alarm is absolutely terrifying, which, I suppose, it should be. It's not just the high-pitched clanging that is bad, but on top of the siren is a loud, male voice shouting that the police have been called. One somewhat amusing comment of the alarm voice is to instruct all burglars to leave the premises. Other than for the alarm, I slept well last night because the medication I take after chemotherapy makes me tired. My fifth treatment was two days ago; only one more to go. Then I begin radiation. Lately I have been having a few dreams about cancer, of the kind that for months were disturbing and recurrent.

January 18, 1988

Since my mastectomy, I have been unable to read the books that people give me about cancer and about coping strategies. These materials simply make the cancer seem real, immediate, and threatening. For example, one well-meaning person sent a rather comprehensive book on various cancers, describing their symptoms, treatments, and prognoses. While I did read the section on breast cancer, I also reviewed parts describing lung and bone carcinomas likely to result from breast cancer metastasis. I was horrified to learn about the treatments and suffering that I might endure if my cancer spread. Now I am trying to read Bernie Siegal's *Love, Medicine, and Miracles*, and a few books describing visualization techniques one might employ while undergoing cancer treatment. According to Siegal, a person could think about chemotherapy drugs as containing little "Pac Man" creatures that eat cancer cells as they course through the veins. I tried these exercises but eventually stopped because I do not like picturing myself with cancer cells. Instead I prefer to work with thoughts of cancer-free blood and tissue and to think about chemotherapy as a cleansing wash.

Gordon is a little upset with me for reading scientific articles about breast cancer. But I am going to read them anyway because I cope better by being informed about my medical condition. He sometimes thinks I am trying to outwit my doctors. Yet the most distressing aspect of my ordeal is feeling out of control, and study of scientific articles helps my need to direct my own destiny. Clearly, there are strong forces in my life that work to limit my sense of free movement and decision, particularly the demands of being married to a university president. Now this added prospect of surrendering my health increases the struggle and creates in me a literal spiritual claustrophobia.

Recently, I found some reports that suggest that first-stage breast cancer recurs at a higher rate than my physicians indicate. One article notes a rate of forty-five percent over an eight-year period: Four of ten first-stage breast cancer patients were dead within eight years. Another argues that mammograms should be discontinued because they do not result in a lower mortality rate for breast cancer patients. Supposedly, mammography only helps detect cancer in earlier stages, so that patients have the illusion they survive longer! More hopeful articles suggest high-survival rates when patients have both chemotherapy and radiation, noting that it has been a fairly common practice not to give first-stage breast cancer patients radiation or chemotherapy. Fortunately, I am treated at a research university where the consensus is that chemotherapy and radiation combined are the appropriate treatment.

Medicine is an inexact science, especially when dealing with cancer. Also disconcerting is realizing the differing results of research findings and the contradictory opinions of physicians. One cancer specialist told me that I could expect a recurrence rate of about thirty-five percent, and another said that a five-to-ten percent recurrence rate was likely. These statistics are presented alongside other complicating variables— the possibility of a new cancer in the opposite breast, the type of surgery one has, and a person's age—all of which place me in a high-risk group.

February 1, 1988

Gordon and I had breakfast together this morning. Hopefully we can spend more time with each other now. More than ever we need to be with each other, in part because we are both still scared about the cancer. And yet our public lives and demanding schedules make evening dates difficult, so we are trying mornings. At 8:30 A.M. we went to a small cafe where we sat at a corner table and hoped no one would recognize us or overhear our conversation.

After breakfast I had some blood drawn. Then I drove into the foothills, just to think and enjoy the scenery. It was snowing lightly and every pine needle was covered with silver. Clouds touched the ground, covering the landscape with shades of white, gray, and gray-blue.

Today I awoke with the thought that I am still alive and am determined to control how I *feel* about this breast cancer even if I cannot master the disease itself. Driving to work, I thought about aspects of this life that I love: brown, dry stipple showing through the snow, ice crystals on branches, rocks gray and round interrupting the smooth expanse of snow. The heat from the car warmed my legs. Gravity pulled me into the seat. How many of these sensations survive death? Will heaven have rushing streams, people who plant gardens?

February 8, 1988

Although I am adjusting to my cancer, it has brought with it a distinct frame of mind, an almost "out-of-body" perspective. My consciousness, now and then, seems to detach from its moorings, and I become a spectator, a watcher of my own life. Sometimes when I am helping Rebekah finish her homework, or I am chairing a meeting or placing a phone call, a new awareness comes over me. I focus upon the stretching tendons in my fingers, the relentless murmur of the overhead fan. I think, "This is amazing to be here, to be touching solid objects, to be hearing these sounds, thinking these ideas." Am I gathering into view a language and symbols that were part of my inner life but not accessible until now?

People go to their jobs. They play with their kids. I wonder what they think. Before I had cancer, I would spend time in seemingly mundane activities: reading a newspaper, outlining a research project, loading the dishwasher. Now I can't go a day without reflection. During my drive to work, then, I look at simple little houses, telephone wires, buildings, lampposts.

February 10, 1988

Morning. I began at 7:45 A.M. with a two-mile walk through the local indoor mall. Last night it snowed and was still snowing when I left the house. The weather obviously discouraged other mall-walkers, and I was completely alone for almost an hour. It is a strange feeling to be somewhere that will become so crowded so soon. Now, however, there is only a mutter of fans. Blue light filters through the skylight and spreads a clean glow on white tiles and tables. Images pass through dark glass and metal grates: a lemon-colored parka, a porcelain doll with stiff yellow hair, sunglasses staring from counter tops. Signs call from many directions at once:

All gold 40% off
On the Move
Energy-ade
For Leasing Information
Special Acrylic Nail
The Excitement is Building at McStain

Finally, Ralph comes, an elderly gentleman who cares for the plants. He wears work pants and a matching baseball cap. Fine gray hair at the nape of his neck curls over his collar. He expresses a certain Edward Hopper forlornness as he sits on a wooden bench and holds a hose into the well while water gushes around the thin trunk of a ficus tree.

Leaving the mall, I feel the cold against my face. When thick snow falls, a strange silence covers the city: Tires spin faintly on the ice; automobile engines hum. Two students laugh as they walk along a sidewalk, the snow creating an acoustic where sound carries indelibly.

February 27, 1988

This weekend the family is at the Broadmoor Hotel in Colorado Springs. I arose before anyone and am sitting in the alcove of our suite.

At first I stayed in bed and looked around the room. "I am alive," I thought to myself, "alive," looking at a queer little light fixture and feeling the texture of the sheet against my neck. I could hear a squirrel chattering, a bird singing.

Now I look out the window at sunlight on magnificent trees, their branches outlined in snow.

February 28, 1988

Is this my dying time? I must learn to die. What is death's lesson? Is it to inform one of life, to throw light on the moment? Without death, would we ponder the mystery of being?

February 29, 1988

I have been thinking of this past weekend, of a swan we saw when we were at the Broadmoor Hotel. It seemed to be dying. I watched it for a long time, transfixed by its graceful, somber pose. The air was bitter cold and sent piercing chills, stiffening the shrubs alongside the hotel's small lake. At the edge of the water, people offered crumbs to hungry ducks and geese. Out in the middle of the ice, far away from other waterfowl, was the swan. It was not dead because I clearly saw it move and preen itself. A leg stretched, then its neck—weighted by its head—arched upward. Then it lowered its beak to a small pool, and drank.

❧ *Bound in a Thin Space*

March 2, 1988

Today I met with the radiologist to plan for treatments that will begin next week. After positioning me on a small, metal table, the doctor drew a grid on my breast and chest and then a dark red line that extended from midpoint on the front of my neck to under my left arm, so that I resembled a map—which is really what I was. My body seemed segmented, like a painted dummy by Léger, wired and glued together. After leaving the hospital, I went shopping, forgetting about the blood-colored line going up my neck—until I noticed that people were staring.

March 6, 1988

Radiation begins on Monday. I have requested a female technician. When I visit the radiation area today to set up the treatment schedule, however, I notice a male technician. On my way out I ask, "Who will be doing my treatment?" The receptionist responds, "Whoever is on duty," meaning it could be the male technician. Latently hysterical, I call Gordon: "I might have a male technician. This is incredible. Not only must I go through what is already a dehumanizing procedure, but I have to worry all the way from Boulder to Denver whether or not I will be greeted by a male technician."

I am angry, but also confused: Am I being overly-sensitive? Is this the way it always is done? I call Gordon; he's angry too, and places a call to the hospital director who is a personal friend. Then I make some calls myself, including one to my nurse friend, Phyllis. "Call Dr. Byyny," she says. "Tell him of your concerns and request a change that makes you comfortable." I am panicking because the radiologist who arranged my treatment is out of town. It is evening, and we still have not reached anyone.

March 7, 1988

In a few hours I begin radiation. Last night the Hospital Administrator called to say he had talked to the Director of Radiation who agreed to arrange for the same woman to do all of my treatments. I was relieved but exhausted from the strain of the ordeal. For days I have been nervous about the procedure because I am uncertain what it will involve. Unlike chemotherapy where injections are every month, radiation will be daily for six weeks. No doubt the continual trips to Denver for treatment, now unaccompanied by Gordon, will be new reminders, reinforcers, of the image of cancer.

At the same time, I am trying very hard to keep some balance in my life and not get overwhelmed by work and unnecessary activities. Fitting two hours for radiation into my daily schedule will not be easy. After today's procedure, I must go to the office and attend committee meetings for the American Cancer Research Center and the Denver Public Schools' Aesthetic Education Institute.

March 8, 1988

I don't know how I can endure these radiation treatments. They are much more difficult than chemotherapy. Whereas chemotherapy involves intrusion of a needle into the arm, this is an invasion of a more private kind. I am not even offered a dressing room and so must disrobe in front of the technician. I must simply enter the treatment room and strip to the waist. On the first day, I spotted a TV monitor that transmitted an image of the radiation table to a monitor sitting in a hall that is frequented by patients, hospital personnel, and others involved with transporting or caring for patients. Immediately, I realized that anyone standing in the hall by the monitor might watch me disrobe if I were near the table. So I found a corner where the camera did not reach, where I could undress out of public view.

March 14, 1988

Radiation again. I hold a white towel in front of me and climb onto a table in a large dark room. Slowly, I press back into gray Styrofoam that has been molded to my head and shoulders. I lie stripped to the waist while an enormous machine spins around me shooting red laser lights across my breast. My reflection—breasts bare, left arm arching over my head—glows from an overhead plate of glass. Protective steel keeps the powerful rays from going outside the targeted area. Around the edge of the treatment room, braced against the wall, are dozens of odd-shaped metal casts of bones, breasts, noses. Outside, hundreds of people stare into a monitor.

March 15, 1988

Today I asked the technician to explain how the monitors are used and why they just sit in the hall of the lab where they can be viewed by anyone who passes. She explains that the monitor is used during treatment to ensure that patients do not move or injure themselves and also that the monitors are in the hall because there is no space for them in other rooms.

"Are the cameras running all the time?" I asked.

"Yes."

"You mean while I am lying on the table or getting ready for treatment, you can see me from the hall?"

"Yes."

"But there was a repairman working on a light fixture right by my monitor."

"Well, we are remodeling and only have room for the monitors in the hall."

"Who else has access to the monitors besides you?"

"Well, other technicians or physicians may view the monitors as a double-checking measure."

"And what about students or other persons passing by the screens?"

"I don't think anyone is particularly interested in looking at the monitors. Students are not normally in the area at the time you are treated, but if they observe you, they will be supervised."

"Will you ask my permission before allowing other observers?"

"That is not our usual procedure."

I dress in my corner and walk from the radiation room. An ambulance driver in a blue shirt sits at my monitor using the screen to fill out a form. When I arrived home, I immediately call Gordon. "This is unbelievably humiliating! They act as though I have no business asking questions, that this is the way it always is and no one else complains." Then I wonder why I yelled at Gordon instead of the radiologist or the technicians. I feel helpless and out of control, dependent upon strangers for life. It is hard to be assertive with cancer health professionals, when they are the only ones who can deliver necessary services. Now I am angry at myself for putting up with this, angry that I did not ask to speak to the radiologist and say that I wouldn't be treated this way. The fact is, I am afraid to want favors, and as a university president's wife, I do not want to assume that I have special powers because this is a university hospital. Yet I feel vulnerable, dependent, unsure, easily led along, it seems, by callous professionals who sorely need to increase the level of their sensitivity.

March 16, 1988

I dread another treatment. On the trip to Denver I think only about monitors. Sometimes I fantasize that I am in a porn film. Fat men with sweaty palms stand around the T.V. screen and gaze into it. I raise my hand over my head. My arm forms a triangle and I feel like the prostitutes posing in Picasso's *Les Demoiselles d'Avignon*, but I am threatened with death if I don't go through this striptease and posturing.

The technician takes Polaroids of my breasts. My face is in the picture too. I turn it to the side and close my eyes, in hope that some University Hospital file clerk does not think, "So this is President Gee's wife." "These are for our records," they say. Who will have access, I wonder, and where will the photographs be kept? Is the cabinet secure? Will they be destroyed or at some time be passed around in research?

Today I finish dressing in the treatment room when a man walks into the room—probably an ambulance driver. He has papers in his hand and is looking for a technician to help him. He pretends not to see me or to observe my startled reflex. People walk in and out all the time. Several times female technicians not involved in my treatment have come into the room while I was on the table, just to get a piece of equipment or ask a question. As I walked from the room, I noticed a man sitting and writing at my monitor.

March 18, 1988

Why am I putting myself through this? Why don't I do something? Take action. Take control. Here I am, someone with supposed expertise in bioethics, in moral principles of "patient autonomy" and "respecting persons," and I am submitting to these indignities. While I do not wish to see myself as overly important, or deserving of more sensitive care than other women, or other patients in general, I do want to believe that there is a standard that should be offered to all and that I am not experiencing it.

March 21, 1988

Gordon is frustrated with my radiation experience and wants to support me. While I feel helpless and would like nothing more than for him to intervene, I must confront this problem myself. It is a way to fight being controlled by the disease. Over the weekend I wrote a letter to the Hospital Director and hand delivered it to his office this morning. Listed were aspects of the procedure that I find humiliating and degrading. He called later and said he was glad I had written, that I had every right to be angry and upset, and that he would call the Radiation Department Chairman and review my concerns. Although I'm glad I took a stand on this issue, I worry that the doctors and hospital administrators will think I am trying to throw my weight around. I even wonder if they will not give me good treatment. Today at radiation, I endured the same indignities, but at least felt I was no longer a passive victim: I had asserted the right to have my human dignity respected.

March 22, 1988

Rebekah is starting to display a certain independence from Gordon and me. Yesterday, she accused us of not understanding her, not sharing her beliefs, nor having anything in common with her. Then she called a friend and told her that we were trying to force her to be like us—boring snobs who do not care about poor people and who only like to go out to dinner and have parties. She attacked me for wearing make-up, for not liking animals or the outdoors, and for being anti-feminist. Undoubtedly, her observations of us had some grain of truth, however painful it was to admit. We do tend to want her to share in our beliefs, we do strike some people as snobs or insensitive. We do have a lot of parties and dinners, we don't have as much time as we wish we had for the outdoors. Sometimes I am too busy or sick to be anyone's friend or keeper or mother. Then Rebekah quickly turns back into her affectionate and loving self. Still I must try to learn from her rather than simply to react with defensiveness or exasperation. I suspect that part of her anger is that my illness and fears are taking their toll in her as well.

I felt a certain guilt and then this evening I saw another side of Rebekah. She had gone to an "etiquette" dinner at church with other youth. They ate spaghetti, with the goal of learning good manners. But

Rebekah said she did not eat much because it kept slipping off her fork. I was still smarting from her criticism of me, when, before falling asleep, Rebekah said she would like to live somewhere other than this boring planet—someplace where there is good shopping.

March 23, 1988

Tonight I am at the law school to catch up on my backlog of work. But Rebekah just called and in a sweet voice told me about a picture she had made.

"I painted three irises," (her favorite flower), she said, and then described their pastel colors.

"Wonderful," I replied. "I'll stop what I'm doing and hurry home to see."

This is the kind of moment I am most grateful for. So I am leaving papers on my desk and rushing out the door.

March 24, 1988

Today was a "down" day. The room where I wait for radiation treatment had just filled with very sick people. Suddenly, a frail black woman went into a seizure and fell from her chair, making a loud cracking noise as her head hit the thinly-carpeted, concrete floor. Probably her cancer had spread to her central nervous system. In some cancers that is what happens: the cancer goes to the bones and then spreads to the central nervous system. Will that be my experience, will I get to the point of seizures? If so, I do not know if I would want to live.

Another man in the room had red ink on his neck from radiology diagrams; obviously, he was very ill because he had to leave the room and recover his strength. Then to my right was a man with red lines on his shaven head. "They removed a tumor the size of a baseball," he said. On my left sat a lively young woman with marks on her cheek who often is there with her husband when I come for treatment. Today she was joking about people staring at her marks in the grocery store. Another strong-looking woman in a light blue jogging suit leaned toward me and said that her breast cancer had spread throughout her lymphatic system. Initially, she had been told she had three months to live, but it was now several years since that diagnosis. "You have to fight cancer," she said.

As I sat trying to concentrate on a book, tears welled in my eyes. Treatment seemed insufferable, and afterward I walked out of the hospital and just kept going in a straight line until I stopped crying.

April 1, 1988

The radiation waiting room is an experience. My favorite patient who comes for treatment is Mr. Witing. He is about thirty years old, faithfully attired in a black leather jacket and black leather top hat—no matter the weather. He wears silver or pewter rings on every finger, thin ones and wider, engraved ones. Attached to his belt is everything, it seems, that was ever important to him—his bottle opener, winter gloves (even on a spring day), keys, and numerous pouches. When he walks, he shuffles and speaks in soft, drawn-out tones. Every day the Red Cross transport service brings him to the hospital. Often I wonder what kind of cancer he has, and if he is going through the experience alone.

Frequently I sit next to a loquacious man who calls me "Boulder" because I drive from Boulder every day. A few months ago, he had a brain tumor but now seems perfectly normal. Another person had surgery on his voice box and speaks in a monotone rasp. A young man in his twenties comes for treatment for lung cancer which was found when a nurse mistakenly sent him for a chest X-ray. On my way to the radiation room, I often pass a man on a stretcher who is waiting for his treatment. He is asleep and hooked to tubes, his skin gray, his cheeks sunken, the flesh around his mouth folding in. One day he seemed alert enough to watch as I passed, and I wondered if I should have smiled and said "hello." After several weeks, I did not see him again.

April 28, 1988

I found a new lump this morning. At least I believe it is new. It is hard to tell, since breast tissue is not perfectly smooth and uniform. Originally, I had a very busy day planned, and now this is all I can think about. I am trying to read a book on "civil religion," but my eyes just sweep back and forth across the page while I remember the recovery room. I call Dr. Robinson. He is out of town today, but can see me tomorrow. He always wants me to come in if I am worried about anything. I know he can sense my terror.

April 30, 1988
(first entry)

Yesterday I had a needle biopsy of the new lump in my breast. The procedure itself was easy by comparison to the reception room waiting and usual pre-test anguish. I remind myself that I have lived through many half-dreams like this, times when I feel only a blur of fear: fear of medical tests, fear of treatments, fear of hospitals, fear of what doctors will say. I had hoped my cancer surgery would end these recurrent traumas, but now I am wondering, will I always find another breast cancer? Will these biopsies and surgeries go on, year after year?

Nurses converse in the hall by the waiting room, patients register at the reception desk. "Do you have your card?" the receptionist asks, then answers the phone, "So he's not feeling well enough to come in?" A young woman sitting next to her husband leafs through a pamphlet on skin cancer and looks up at me: I know that she is wondering what kind I have. I try reading, drum my fingers, then close my eyes. I start editing papers, but my thoughts won't focus. My pen is heavy in my hand. A few days of waiting, and these few moments before I see the doctor, feel like years.

Now everything is over. Dr. Robinson says I am okay. I feel a great sense of relief but know I still have a distance to go to heal psychologically and spiritually from my cancer, and so does Gordon. For several days this past week Gordon was away. It was the first time he had been by himself long enough to really reflect deeply on his feelings. When he called, he said that it was hard to be alone in the hotel room with nothing to do but think about what life for Rebekah and him would be like without me.

April 30, 1988
(second entry)

I have hardly written in my journal this month, and it felt so good to write this morning that I returned to it again this evening. Journal writing is normally my outlet for creativity and, more importantly, a way for shaping abstract feelings into clear thoughts. But I notice that when I feel emotionally overwhelmed the writing stops. Radiation seems to be numbing my mind so I almost have to force myself to put words on a page.

A couple of doctors affiliated with the Radiation Department did speak to me about my complaints: A male physician was sympathetic and said he would reevaluate their procedures in light of my concerns. Then a female doctor in charge of the lab visited with me before one of my treatments, indicating that she had been made aware of my criticism. She made excuses about the monitors being in the hall and said it was hard to tell ambulance drivers what to do. I didn't really expect anything to change overnight and nothing really has. The monitors are still in the corridor; I still hover in the corner of the treatment room to undress, men in blue work shirts still pass by the monitors, but stopping my treatments is not one of my choices.

May 2, 1988
(first entry)

I underestimated the time and effort it takes to drive to Denver each day, see doctors, have blood tests. Initially, I anticipated finishing my treatments and getting to the office by 9:30 A.M. Instead it is 11:30 A.M. when I arrive at the office, and I have to leave by 4:00 P.M. Consequently, my work is piling up because I simply lack time and energy to get it done. Then, too, I am emotionally exhausted from the ongoing humiliation of the procedure. After my surgeries, I worked very hard to institute a daily schedule that allows for personal development—writing in my journal, reading, exercising, being of small service to anyone, doing physical therapy for my back, finding a few quiet moments with Gordon. Now I have had to abandon almost all of these, which makes me feel very out of control at a time I need to feel in charge of my life.

May 2, 1988
(second entry)

Radiation is making me think about death every day, but I am not coming to profound conclusions. In fact, I'm amazed that things associated with cancer so frequently interrupt my daily thoughts. In truth, I am glad that I have time to reflect upon it, and that death has not come upon me by surprise. What lies ahead after life? Will there be microwave ovens, word processors, answering machines? I realize that I am being whimsical, but there is a certain point in these wanderings, a certain instruction. Is this the only time I will take a hot shower, smell lilacs, eat curry? I try sharing some of these thoughts with Gordon, but he does not connect with much that I say: He admits that he never thinks such things. Sometimes it seems that he could be suffering a kind of denial, unwilling to confront notions and innuendoes— however tongue-in-cheek—about death. This may be a way of affirming his love for me. Still, I wish we could talk.

May 3, 1988

Radiation is finally over and already I feel life returning to me. Today, almost eight months after my surgery, I write in my journal, and, in a few minutes, will walk in the field. Then I will work on a paper that I will present at Indiana University in the fall which will focus on religious ideals underlying professional volunteerism. All day I have been thinking that I have surmounted a major hurdle, that the course of my psychological and spiritual progress which seemed detoured during radiation can now follow a more direct route. Thoughts of dying still flash through my mind virtually every hour of the day, sometimes when I least expect them—in the middle of a telephone conversation, while combing my hair, or during a meeting. Lying in bed at night, trying to go to sleep, is when the most disturbing specters haunt the darkness of my room: I.V. tubes, a wall rising between my family and me, the murmuring of loved ones gathered around the bed, my gaunt face contorted by pain and morphine. Still these images, horrifying as they are, are less unsettling than they once were in the weeks following surgery. Now they don't stay with me all day and sometimes all night as they did then. I have grown to expect a few ghosts to hover as I drift off to sleep, and I'm no longer alarmed at their presence. In fact, these bedtime apparitions, rather than frightening me, now prompt thoughts about belief in God, and forms of spiritual life that continue past death. A week ago, an elderly friend died, and I thought all day about what he must be experiencing and how beautiful and extraordinary the event of death is. Perhaps the difference between my feelings now and several months ago is this: I am as captivated by the wonder of death as by the fear of death.

ॐ Returning to the Question

May 8, 1988

Last night, Gordon, Rebekah, and I attended the opera, *Carmen*, in Denver. Rebekah wore a new dress—light blue with white flowers—made especially for the occasion. Her blonde hair was pulled into a horizontal French braid, and a small row of pearls rested on her neck. Finally, a beauty-shop manicure made bitten nails look surprisingly good, and a touch of make-up gave her skin a warm glow. No one could question that she looked beautiful and very grown-up.

Totally enthralled by the music and staging, Rebekah sang the songs all the way home to Boulder even though it was 1:00 A.M. Gordon and I also enjoyed the performance, although a book I read as a child, *Otis Spofford*, forever ruined the "Toreador" song. Whenever I listen to music from *Carmen*, I hear Otis sing: "Toreador-a, Don't spit on the floor-a, Use a cuspidor-a, That's what it's for-a." I imagine this sensation means that my sense of humor is returning.

May 12, 1988

I went home at noon today to help host a luncheon for commencement honorees, about forty people, several of whom are to be recognized tomorrow at various graduation ceremonies. On the way, I thought about this time of passage in the life of a university and felt grateful at being alive to experience it once again. It was a bright, sunny day, so I walked onto the patio for a view of the mountains and to enjoy the beauty of the day. Our perspective of the Flatirons is almost unique in Boulder because the home is set back in a field, far enough that we also see the higher, snowy Rocky Mountains. The Flatirons rise over graceful meadows and spring grasses, above ridges of stone and pine. Birds lift off from a tree near the house and throw a screen of black against the sky.

This is Gordon's favorite time of the academic year, probably because it affirms who he is professionally, and today he was in particularly good form. I enjoyed watching him mingle with our guests, congratulating them on their achievement or chatting with them about the glorious weather.

One of our guests today was actor and alumnus, Robert Redford. He will be receiving an honorary doctorate for his environmental work and support of young film companies.

Mr. Redford was one of the first to arrive at our home for lunch and was standing on the front step conversing with Gordon when a car approached with an elderly woman whose husband was being honored at commencement by the university. Soon the car pulled around the circle of the front drive and parked right in front of Mr. Redford. Instinctively, he swept down the steps and opened the passenger door. The look on this woman's face was one of disbelief when she recognized Robert Redford holding her door open and waiting to escort her into the house. I sat next to him at lunch and felt a new sense of awareness of the moment and its details: the saffron-colored veins radiating from white flowers in the center of the table, the wide eyes of a young woman on my right, the blend of voices that swelled between each luncheon course, the tattered friendship bracelet around Mr. Redford's wrist.

May 13, 1988

Today was commencement at the University of Colorado at Boulder. I did not attend the entire ceremony, but just the beginning, so that I could hear Gordon speak. The students always give him a warm reception, often standing or applauding as the procession of dignitaries and faculty passes. Frequently, he stops to shake their hands or, once in awhile, give a "high five" to an exuberant student. For many years I have attended spring commencement. The students walk lightly. Their black silk robes bubble in the wind as they circle gardens, dodge cars, stop to joke with friends, and have pictures taken with parents beside the bronze Buffalo.

Like Gordon, I am always renewed by graduation and feel a sense of completion that another year is drawing to a close. "Pay day," one university regent says. From the time I was eleven and my mother worked at the University of Utah, my life has been geared to the academic calendar. Since then, I have not been away from a university campus. The seasons of college life are an aspect of my personal rhythm.

Gordon spoke about me and my cancer surgery in his commencement address, inviting the students to integrity and self-confidence, and to cultivate personal resources of family and friends to sustain them in times of crisis. As I walked away from the Events Center, I looked at the mountains, the gray-rose stone of the Flatirons.

May 25, 1988

Some women faculty members joined me at the university residence for lunch. Nancy Hill, a faculty member in the Humanities Department, and Mary Ann Shea, the Director of the Excellence in Teaching program at the university, and I started a support group for faculty women—an informal get-together where we can meet to develop a sense of friendship and community. We feel that women are still marginalized within university settings and that traditional departments can be very limiting in the opportunities that they provide for exchange among academic women. Over the past months, the group has evolved in essentially the way that we had anticipated, as a means for free, informal, and supportive sharing of ideas. Even though we have met just a few times, I feel a growing sense of attachment to these women and am fed by their creativity, intellect, and personal compassion.

The cultural expectations of the role of a university president's spouse are changing, thank goodness, so I felt free to form such a group. Today there are other ways of supporting universities besides teas and dinner parties. My personal approach is to create programs and not simply serve as a kind of social ambassador. Some wives are involved totally with their president husbands' commitments, others are a bit defiant, and a few choose to be totally uninvolved with university matters—particularly those women who have demanding professions. While my professional work and scholarly interests remain important to me, I believe in education and feel that these years married to a university president offer many rare opportunities to make a contribution to society.

June 2, 1988

Gordon and I had breakfast together this morning. We had a very intimate conversation about what we would do in the event that either of us died. Our talk was both painful and loving. We felt neither of us would remarry, and the surviving spouse would work hard to keep memories of the other alive. This was an important agreement for me. Deep inside, I am afraid I will be forgotten when I die. I fear this probably because I do not retain many memories of my father; I feel I have forgotten him. Then we talked about Rebekah and ways to ensure her support in the event one of us should die. Truthfully, there would be more disruption to Rebekah's lifestyle if Gordon were to die because we would have to move from the university-owned home and eventually lose many university-related advantages, services, and perhaps even ties with people who have become significant in our lives. I feel better now that we have had this talk.

June 14, 1988

This past week, Rebekah and I spent a lively time in New York City. It was wonderful having several uninterrupted days just to be together. I can tell that I have made good emotional progress since my last trip to New York in December. Then I felt almost desperate about going with Gordon and Rebekah, and I thought constantly about death and dying no matter what we were doing. This time I was already in New York for a Hastings Center Board of Directors meeting. The Hastings Center is an ethics "think tank" in New York, and I have served on their board for several years. On Friday the meetings concluded and that evening Rebekah flew to meet me. Although Rebekah loves New York, she has not had an opportunity to visit the city during the summer. For the most part, our New York family trips have been in December, so there is a big part of the city she has not seen—Central Park, the Fountain at Rockefeller Center, the Upper West Side, Soho—places that are not inviting in cold temperatures and high winds.

Seeing the David Hockney exhibit at the Metropolitan Museum of Art was one of the principal objectives of our trip. One way I have worked to cultivate Rebekah's aesthetic sensibilities and interests is to take her to art shows, hoping she will fall in love with art as I did many years ago. Soon after moving to Colorado, when she was ten, we drove to Santa Fe to see a retrospective of Georgia O'Keeffe's paintings. Although it was a short excursion, our time together was good, and we learned a lot about O'Keeffe. The exhibit ranged from her early realistic works to the large flower abstracts. Quickly, Rebekah picked out favorites in the show and even seemed to appreciate the stylized flowers, clouds, and New Mexico landscape. Standing next to an elderly couple who were making an, "I could have painted that myself" observation, Rebekah turned and said, "Some people just don't understand art." It seems to me that the progression of a child's awareness and interest in art is not automatic, but rather a slow evolution. For a long time, Rebekah did not like what she termed "flat art," but preferred sculpture and kinetic objects. Then she also seemed blind to scenery and to the aesthetics of nature, but now I notice she is changing and that she often points out cloud formations and mountain streams.

June 16, 1988

In a few hours, Rebekah, Gordon, and I leave for San Diego where Gordon has a meeting. I came to the law school office this morning to have a few minutes of peace and quiet to write in my journal and work on a report prepared for the Center for Health Ethics and Policy, an assignment which has brought a certain pressure in recent weeks. Without much warning, I was given the task of compiling and synthesizing some survey results. Recently, the Center surveyed Colorado physicians as to their views on terminating life-sustaining treatment. Not surprisingly, the findings suggest that physicians do not think that life should be prolonged, and some even acknowledge giving assistance to patients to commit suicide. The report, when released, made a big splash with the press, and I had to spend too many hours in press conferences and with news reporters.

Sometimes I think about what I would want in the final stages of terminal illness. I know that I want to preserve my sense of control and not be totally dependent upon others, especially family. That is, I would not want to lose all my privacy and dignity by having others take me to the bathroom, bathe me, and clothe me. And if I cannot do these things myself, I would prefer a professional nurse to assist me, someone I do not know too well, so that there would be a certain protection, a certain anonymity. I have a way of being with Gordon and Rebekah that must not be transformed, so that I become, in essence, their "child." Even in death and dying, I want to continue as wife and mother. Should I become incapacitated and incompetent to make important health decisions, my family should make the decisions that best satisfy their needs. Although I would prefer to have some dignity in my last days and not become someone who is unrecognizable to ones I love, dying is not a singular process. Others share in the experience and must live with the memories.

June 27, 1988

More and more I find myself wishing we could live in a private home rather than a university residence. This is probably because my cancer has made me feel a greater need for privacy and personal time with Gordon and Rebekah. This week we have four public functions to host, three to be held at our home. For a good portion of every day, the family relinquishes its home to other people—housekeepers, caterers, grounds crews, repair persons. Often we feel compelled to leave our home, to get out of their way so they can accomplish their work. If we are ill, or if there are things at home that we need to work on, we are intruders. Typically, the requisite parties and social gatherings take several days worth of preparation and require that normal family evening activities be suspended. Last year Gordon and I hosted seventy functions, over forty at our home. It is not unusual for us to invite as many as three or four thousand people to the residence in a nine-month period. Yet the most painful consequence of living in such a residence is having those we entrust with personal matters, who help care for our child, or who are so close that they know intimate details of our personal lives, betray us. Many wonderful people have worked with our family, and in a way become part of the family, but there have also been those who tried to undermine Gordon and me with Rebekah, who stole from us, or who tried to tarnish our reputation within the university. Public life has an element of invasiveness that sometimes feels like doctors have stripped off your clothes and cut into your flesh.

Despite these inconveniences and hazards, there is wisdom in making the president's residence public. Besides the support it provides the family—a rent-free place to live and space for performing the duties a president has in fund-raising and in receiving university visitors—there is symbolic value. The symbolism of "home" and the personal spirituality of our family strikes a chord with visitors and those who would support the university, perhaps because knowledge begins and is perhaps most profound at the home and family level.

June 29, 1988

Although we have been living in the university residence since last July, my illness has made it difficult to complete the finishing touches. Now I must take time to work out the bugs, and we have an infestation of them: The plumbing was installed backwards, catering kitchen appliances block ventilation systems, the chimney flues blow smoke into entertaining areas, and the roof leaks into the living room. This summer the landscaping will receive some needed attention, and hopefully some trees and other shrubbery can be planted as protection to the house from the raging Boulder chinooks—or high winds from the mountains—that sometimes exceed one hundred miles per hour. It is impossible to sleep in the master bedroom when winds pound our west walls—they rage against the damper, and the windows shake so hard that I lie awake fearing they will blow out. A few nights ago, the windstorm was so fierce that I simply could not sleep. Finally, at four in the morning, I climbed into bed with Rebekah, because her room is the most protected from these storms. She has an antique brass bed that sits quite high off the floor, and as I lay there trying to go to sleep, I could hear a loud rhythmic squeaking. Then I realized that the winds were coming at the house so forcefully that the whole structure was shaking, and Rebekah's rather fragile bed had been set in motion.

July 5, 1988

Gordon, Rebekah, and I are on a week-long vacation in Santa Fe where we are staying at the Inn on the Alameda, a nice bed and breakfast hotel that serves exquisite fruit and rolls every morning. Because the room offers a wonderful view of the surroundings, at sunset we stand on the deck and watch the sagebrush and sand turn red and orange and a luscious sky become purple and gray. And for the past few days, we have been real tourists, visiting the museums, the Governor's Palace, and so many art galleries that Rebekah now protests about seeing more. Yesterday we attended a Fourth of July pancake breakfast at the city plaza, where we listened to the band and walked through an antique car show. Then, at night, we watched fireworks from the hood of our car in the local high school parking lot.

Every morning, starting early because the sun quickly becomes unbearably hot, Gordon and I walk. We explore the downtown area on foot, passing unique pink and brown adobes, people watering their lawns, and street merchants setting out wares. Occasionally, we stop to get Rebekah a breakfast treat. She sleeps while we are gone, although sometimes she awakens and is watching cartoons when we arrive back at the Inn.

These brief excursions give us needed time to talk. While I believe my recovery from cancer surgery has been positive and steady, I know from the articles I read that spouses of cancer victims often have greater and more long-term distress than do the patients. From my own experience, I can see why this is the case, since I, and not Gordon, am checked by the doctors on a regular basis. I know the mortality statistics that pertain to my case; I had volunteers from cancer associations counsel with me about my disease, and I had time to address the issue of dying and what it means for me and my family. In essence, I have a greater sense of understanding and control of the situation. Gordon, on the other hand, has had little time even to think about what my cancer means to him. Probably this realization is what finally hit him a few months ago when he was out of town and alone in a hotel room. Perhaps he feels some guilt for the times he did not take my fears about breast cancer very seriously, or that he could not stop the degradation I experienced with the radiation treatments. As much as we both hoped that his work could slow down a bit, universities are demanding institutions that don't make allowance for personal crisis. So, even in the days and weeks following my surgery, Gordon had to maintain his normal work schedule, which on a good week allows for dinner at home only three nights with the other four days a week stretching into fourteen-hour days. In many respects, he knows he is helpless: He can't guarantee that the cancer won't return, he can't be there to keep me company, do the housework when I am tired, or help Rebekah with her homework. As I think about these pressures for him, I can better understand the changes in our marital relationship over the past months. I know we both feel a new love for each other and oneness in our relationship that is deep and abiding, so much so that sometimes I think I can read his thoughts by the way he glances out the window or wrinkles his brow; yet, there are times when I feel isolated from him, when the communication between us seems awkward and forced. Sometimes when we have scheduled time together, such as this trip, there is so much silence that I wonder if being with me is hard on him and whether my presence calls up hurtful images and fears.

July 13, 1988

On July 8 we left Santa Fe to drive to Durango. On our route were old Western towns that stretched along narrow gray roads and railroad tracks and yellow flowers which softened the expanse of sage and weed. Following a path of asphalt through clusters of sullen shacks, we saw mountains, cliffs the color of red and gold, and forest-covered peaks sinking into deep canyons.

At about 4:30 P.M. we arrived in Durango. Several messages were awaiting Gordon, including one from Malcolm Justice, his brother-in-law. I had forgotten that today was when Gordon's father was undergoing an angioplasty, a procedure to open his clogged arteries and heart valve.

"I'd better call him," Gordon said. "I hate messages like this."

"You had better call."

Then I heard Gordon cry out. His father had died. Over and over every day, this sound still recurs in my mind. Rebekah was in the room when the news came. She was very sweet and concerned. We said a prayer, and then Gordon left to go for a drive in the car by himself. Later we ordered room service for dinner and then walked around the town a bit. So that Gordon could have some time to himself, I took Rebekah to a movie, but I was in a daze the whole time. I think one of the reasons I married Gordon was because of his father. Even now, I remember the first day I met Gordon's parents, how his father held his mother's hand, how he carefully listened when she talked, how he brightened when she told a story about her father. Faithfully, he treated his wife with love and compassion, and I knew Gordon would follow in his ways.

July 17, 1988

We have just returned from Gordon's father's funeral. The day after learning of his death, we drove straight from Durango to Boulder. Then we hurriedly packed our bags and flew to Salt Lake the following morning. Gordon's father had been suffering from a deteriorated hip and weak heart and had undergone the angioplasty in preparation for hip surgery. We knew there was some risk, but just had not anticipated that he would die during the procedure from a tear in the artery. In Salt Lake we learned that Malcolm had a premonition of his death and even returned to the hospital room to tell Gordon's father that his family loved him.

I know Gordon still is in shock and is trying to comprehend that his father is gone. I think constantly about his dad: All day, memories flash by of him holding Rebekah in his arms when she was three-weeks old; sitting on the patio at the home of Gordon's sister, Cherie; his telling a joke and then laughing before anyone else had a chance to; and admonishing Gordon to "Be good. You know the rules." When I think about the way he died, I wonder if there is a best speed for dying. The quick death seems harsh, unfair, depriving loved ones of a chance to say goodbye; the protracted death leaves time for closure but often makes the dying person and his or her family extend their suffering and grief.

I would rather die a quick death than one that is drawn out in the way terminal cancer can be, but I guess I am more afraid of the process of dying than of death itself, and research indicates that most people feel the same way. Probably, Gordon's father would have preferred to go quickly, perhaps the way he did, rather than suffer what assuredly would have been a lingering decline. The funeral was held at the chapel where

Gordon's father and mother attended church. Many people came. Family members spoke, including Gordon. Then Gordon's dad was buried in a beautiful patch of green, alongside the road that he had traveled weekly to his daughter's home for Sunday dinner.

July 19, 1988

I have been thinking about Gordon's father, wondering how it was for him when he left this world and if leaving has much to do with readiness. Hamlet suggests this when likening his own inevitable death to the "special providence in the fall of a sparrow. If it be now, 'tis not to come; if it be not to come, it will be now; if it be not now, yet it will come. The readiness is all," Hamlet concludes.

Am I more ready than I was a year ago because I've had a chance to consider the question? Yes, I think so. While a separation from so much I love remains incomprehensible, still I feel a deep reassurance that there is great continuity between this earth and the life we will find when we go.

August 5, 1988

It has been several weeks since my last journal entry, and I miss my personal writing. Gordon, Rebekah, and I have been vacationing in Breckenridge since Monday. Mainly we are trying to relax, read, and enjoy each other. Yesterday we hiked to the waterfall in McCulloch's Gulch, beginning at the base of 14,000-foot Quandary Peak and climbing 1,000 feet in a mere mile and a half. Our hearts pounded as we drew thin air into our lungs and made our way along a soft, pine-needle path. No matter how slowly we walked or how deeply we breathed, there never seemed to be enough oxygen, so we stopped often to throw pebbles in the stream, peel transparent layers of mica stones, and study an abundance of wildflowers which bear a remarkable diversity of color this year. Dropping from one narrow ledge was a steep embankment covered with indigo, ultramarine, reddish purple, pinks, yellows, and pale lavenders, with rocks, wild grass, and veins of rich black soil.

Rebekah has done quite a bit of baking since we have been here in Breckenridge—gold-rush brownies, scones, corn bread, and fudge. She bakes, and we eat. Tonight I am putting prints in the photo album, a task I have been wanting to complete for months. It seems I save the photographs for so long that often I cannot remember when or why I took them. There are more photographs of quaint European towns in these albums than I will ever be able to identify.

It is raining now, and the drops make pools of circling lines in the pond. The rain shears through the pine needles onto the shuddering willows, and sounds of thunder mix with the relentless roaring of the stream.

August 6, 1988

Breckenridge. I still think about my cancer daily and about how long I will live. I must find a greater sense of peace about life and death. To fully experience this life is what matters, to find what Hannah Arendt called "consciousness of consciousness." Eternity is now, here today as much as at the edge of death. I seek one thing, to see purely the brightness of my humanity.

August 7, 1988

The sun has dropped behind the mountain facing our Breckenridge home and is no longer visible. Only one small cluster of clouds floats just above the pines and glows a blinding white. From a window I see the pond which shimmers now with slices of silver evening sky. Today I sat on the bank of the stream, balancing myself on an uncomfortable triangle of rock, and watched the water descend several hundred feet, cascading freely along the path it made years ago. I think about the volume of water that passes in just one day, how many times the water in the pond is displaced—perhaps thousands.

Cool air is starting to come through the three-inch opening in the window by the table where I am writing while indoor and outdoor lights—warm gold and soft gray—enhance the texture of the table's wood grain. This piece of furniture belonged to my great, great, grandmother, Rachel Ridgeway Ivins Grant. Several years ago, my mother's older sister, Rachel, gave it to me because she knew I liked old things. So many stories are in this table, lives etched in its solid walnut leaves and sturdy turned legs which rest on rather fragile-looking porcelain coasters.

I remember the table from when my mother, brother, and I lived with Grandma and Grandpa Cannon after my father died. The table stood in the laundry room in the basement, a large space with a painted gray concrete floor and a variety of laundry equipment: mangle, wash tubs, a wringer washing machine, scrub board and electric washer and dryer—all this and Grandma still hung the laundry on the backyard clothes line. As far as I remember, the table did not serve any particular purpose, although Mother says it was sometimes used for ironing. Obviously, girls used it for sewing, which I can tell from marks left by the teeth of a metal tracing wheel used to inscribe seam lines with carbon paper. On both ends of the straight planks are grooves from something that was tightly clamped, perhaps an apple peeler or meat grinder. These scars are deep and black, showing constant use and intense pressure. Another set of regularly-spaced marks could have been left by a small boy pounding something on the table, and a round, black burn was likely left by a candle or an upended iron. Over the years, sections of the wood have been replaced, so that parts of the table are lighter. Now I am making my own contribution to the heritage of this piece—scrape marks from the laptop computer, stains from spilled beverages, and scratches from dishes and utensils.

It is rare, when I sit at this table, that I do not think about its first owner: The family refers to her as Grandma Grant. Aunt Rachel and Mother knew her when they were growing up because she lived with Grandma and Grandpa Cannon and their children until her death. Apparently, she was a fastidious woman whose appearance was impeccable and who kept her small attic room immaculately clean. She had been a widow most of her life and developed many ways of being self-sufficient, including crocheting handkerchiefs and doing fine needle work. I'm lucky to have one of her handkerchiefs, its edges the finest, most delicate work of crocheting I have ever seen.

August 10, 1988

Gordon and I are staying in the mountains this week while Rebekah goes to church camp. All day we sit on the deck and read, listen to the stream, smell the fresh pines. Right now I am starting Thomas Hardy's *Far from the Madding Crowd* and just finished *Beloved*, by Toni Morrison—a powerful book. Also I brought along a biography of Pablo Picasso and two books about modern theories of physics: Stephen Hawking's *A Brief History of Time* and James Gleick's *Chaos*. For years I have been fascinated by physics, including recent attention to the "new physics," string theory, and chaos theory, although I do not pretend to understand equations. Physics to me is like mythology and religion, great stories that explain the mystery of life. Yet as I read, the text seems that it grasps at a reality to which only a few have access.

August 14, 1988

This life often seems a brief summer vacation, a trip to places where we see new things. Or occasionally, mortal life strikes me as foreign—even contradictory to the rest of being. Sometimes the trees, cars, houses, shopping centers seem irrelevant, even a debasement of the poetry of existing, or I get irritated spending time running to the drugstore or tidying the kitchen after dinner. It seems hard to sustain profound thought when we must expend so much energy on mundane routine.

Perhaps the answer is in trying to appreciate the concreteness and meaning of apparent trifles; seeing their connection, or contribution, to the continuity and constancy of all life—both immortal and mortal aspects: beauty even in a dead tree, half submerged in a pond; beauty as small as a grasshopper clinging to its branches; and beauty beyond a fussing child—to a child's soul.

August 26, 1988

Today is our twentieth wedding anniversary. Gordon and I have been celebrating in San Francisco and Carmel. Our honeymoon was a trip to Lake Tahoe, San Francisco, and Carmel, so we thought it would stir our nostalgia or excite an old sense of new life to return to the same area. Rebekah is vacationing at Lake Powell with Gordon's sister, Cherie, her husband, Malcolm, and other family members. For a few days we stayed at a charming bed and breakfast hotel, the White Swan Inn, which is located atop a very steep hill. While there, we shopped, dined, browsed through Fisherman's Wharf and Ghiradelli Square, and in the mornings donned our tennis shoes and walked the town. We vowed to return in another twenty years—just to see if we could still make it up the steep streets.

After our four-day visit to San Francisco, we drove along Route 1, following the coastline, to Carmel. Once there, we relaxed, read, slept late, browsed through stores. On a clear day we took a picnic lunch and drove the seventeen-mile road through the Pebble Beach area. Sitting on a ragged log, we watched the waves roll and gulls sway above in the ocean breeze. For a while we talked about our wedding day and the early years of marriage; our first impressions upon moving to New York as newly-weds, and when we drove through the New York City cemetery that seemed to go on for miles and through narrow roads faced by angry-looking buildings; how in setting up housekeeping in a one-bedroom student apartment, we never envisioned lives we now lead; our some-times exhausting but always stimulating involvement in universities; and the joy we share in having a child.

September 14, 1988

One year ago today I underwent breast cancer surgery. As the anniversary of my surgery has approached, my mind has been filled with memories: the physical trauma of surgery, the shock of the word *cancer*, and feeling out of control. This past year has been important, for I have learned much and matured in ways I never thought possible. I am a different person now. Assuredly, I do not want to return to my old self. I guess I am thankful it all happened. In an important sense, cancer is a calling, a calling to adventure that if accepted culminates in the passage to a new humanity and an even greater understanding of the wonder of life. The other response, the other view of cancer or any crisis—that rejects the call, that refuses to look for meanings, other sorts of wellness, and possibilities—transforms the potential adventure into a disaster, a void, a state where promise and hope are relinquished, and where the protagonist is a victim.

I have a new sense of being with Gordon and Rebekah and of loving them. I notice the smoothness of Rebekah's skin, the pleasure of being able to wrap my arm around her waist, or loop my fingers through hers. Or I feel Gordon's warmth against me as I struggle to sleep. Simply, I am recognizing the fine details of life, seeing through a magnifying lens to the figures of the "lived life" that Maurice Merleau-Ponty talks about. When I walk, I am conscious of the wind on my face. Holding a leaf, I notice its texture and temperature. However long I live, daily life now has a richness that has to do with love.

This past year I have sought to identify life's great themes, what we are about as humans, how I might fully experience being alive, what opportunities might be seized now, and what dimensions of living in this world might be eternal. What categories and patterns signify life in its entirety? It is a big task to master these issues, but such a quest has already helped me to better reflect on the constants of virtue, knowledge, community, family, charity, faith, obedience, diligence—qualities that Joseph Campbell, the renowned mythologist, might have called an order of eternity, clues to an inner divinity that can be experienced and utilized at every moment. The questions raised by cancer and the prospect of death are torchlights of truth that illuminate unknown bends on a dark road. So now I know better how to live in this world, and where to spend time. Every morning I open on joy, each day I discover much to love.

I also have a new sense of oneness with God, although it is not as strong as I would like. I still do not have the feeling I am seeking: a sense of peace, or assurance that no matter the course of events, everything is all right.

This evening at dusk Gordon and I walked along Caddo Parkway, the road in front of our house. As we circled the pond at Thunderbird Park, mountains were reflected in the water, and black swamp birds with red epaulets darted among the reeds. When we returned, Gordon went into the house, and I sat by the fountain in our back yard, watching the sky grow dark and the lights in the garden gradually begin to illuminate the vegetation. Rebekah was inside with her friend, Eva. I feel a peace now, a certainty that there is truth which stretches forever from one crest of life to the next, and that there is nothing to fear in life or death.

September 21, 1988

I found an enlarged lump in my right breast last night and immediately knew I was in trouble. This one was different from the small lesions that have surfaced since the mastectomy. There had been something small there for a while, but it increased in size during the last month. I noticed it while taking a shower. Gordon was already in bed, starting to go to sleep, when I slipped between the sheets and moved close to him. Then I told him what I had found. It did not seem possible that I would keep having problems after the subcutaneous mastectomy. After all, the surgeon said that he had removed ninety-five percent of the breast tissue. Didn't that eliminate the risk of a second cancer? Gordon pulled me near, and I started to cry—at first quietly but soon with racking sobs. I cried uncontrollably, as never before, so loudly that Gordon got up and closed the bedroom door to keep from waking Rebekah. The specter of last year rose before me, and I could feel the cancer in my flesh, feel the unbearable pressure against my chest. Suddenly, I was reliving the worst moments of my terror. The faces, smells, pokes, X-rays rushed in like a wave. Finally, the images grew smaller, and I felt a certain anger or embarrassment at my breakdown.

September 23, 1988

I saw Dr. Robinson today, and he performed a needle aspiration. Gordon went with me to give moral support. "The results will not be available for a couple of hours," he said. "I will call you as soon as I get the report. I want to look at the slides myself."

Gordon and I walked to the elevators.

"Shall we go for a drive? We could get something to eat," Gordon said.

"Let's ride for a while," I replied.

There is not a lot that will remove the anxiety of such waiting, but being with Gordon helps. We head toward Boulder, but instead of taking the usual route follow the interstate toward Ft. Collins. Once out of Denver, the road cuts through wide expanses of green farmland and pastures. It is a pleasant route, where sleek black angus graze on green, and the sky makes a wide arch over the plains. But mostly I think about the test results. We stop at McDonald's for a drink, then go home, so that we will not miss the call.

When we pull into the garage, the housekeeper says, "A Dr. Robinson has been calling. He said he must speak to Elizabeth or Gordon." There is an urgency in her voice that is unsettling, a tenseness in her glance. I want her to leave—I want privacy, to be alone. Gordon and I go upstairs to the bedroom where no one will disturb us. I think about all of the waiting I have done over the past twenty years, not being able to go more than six months or a year without a lesion or cyst developing that we need to watch. This ghost is coming again: Those nights will be here when I can't sleep, when I won't eat, when the boundaries of life will reappear.

Gordon sits at the desk and dials the number. I stand watching for a few seconds, but my legs won't hold. I lie down on the floor by the fireplace, roll onto one side, and pull my legs to my chest. "Bill, this is

Gordon," then silence. I rise to my knees and search Gordon's eyes. He is staring at the desk. After a few "uh-huhs," Gordon hands the phone to me.

"The needle biopsy is really inconclusive, Elizabeth," Dr. Robinson says. "I estimate about a fifty percent chance of malignancy. Even with the subcutaneous mastectomy you still have some remaining breast tissue that is vulnerable to a second cancer. We will do a biopsy first thing next week."

September 24, 1988

I attended a session today at the Mormon temple in Denver. I thought it might help ground my feelings of the last couple of days, and it did. Almost immediately upon entering the building, I felt a peace that seemed held in a reassuring, transcendent spirit. I am sorry for people who must live through their fears without a similar kind of resource. It must be difficult to feel pressure building, when your body has sealed in bad dreams, and you have no ready way to set them free.

September 26, 1988

All weekend Gordon and I have been on the phone with doctors, discussing various scenarios as to the outcome of the biopsy tomorrow. If it is malignant, I will undergo a full bilateral mastectomy, an operation to remove the implants and all remaining breast tissue before the end of the week. Pictures I have seen of women who have lost their breasts to crescent-shaped scars pass through my dreams, but I don't have time to focus on these images. Our lives are so busy that it even seems impossible that we should have to drop everything and check into the hospital for surgery. Gordon will have to clear his calendar, and I will make other plans for my work and Rebekah's care. A few months ago, I called my mother and alerted her, so that she could fly out to be with Rebekah. We did not want to say anything to Rebekah about the possibility of cancer, but we did tell her about the biopsy. One night, when putting her to bed, we talked about the health problems that I have had and

what certain procedures were or would be like. She was very understanding and seemed relieved to know what our tense body language
had expressed.

Now I am thinking about all the preparations I need to make: I must
go over Rebekah's calendar, see that my meetings are canceled, answer
important mail, and review drafts of my paper for Indiana University.
Last night I reminded Gordon where I keep my journal, so that it
would not get thrown away should I not survive the operation. I called
Phyllis and told her what was happening. We talked for a while, and
she said she would fly out from South Carolina to be with me if I had
surgery. I count the hours until we get into the car and drive to the
University Hospital. "The biopsy will be over by this time tomorrow," I
tell myself. Then I will know.

September 27, 1988

The biopsy is over. The lump was not malignant. Dr. Ketch—the
plastic surgeon who performed my first cancer operation—did the
procedure while Dr. Byyny held my hand and Dr. Robinson assisted.
The procedure was quick and painless. I did not have any sedation, and
the four of us conversed and joked, mainly about university football,
during the brief procedure. The pathologist immediately examined
the specimen, and I had a clean bill of health within an hour after
arriving at the hospital. Gordon and I were jubilant! We visited with
the doctors and then went to our car where we could cry.

October 3, 1988

Today I am in New York to help with some university fund raising.
The main purpose of the trip is to have dinner with Robert Lee
Morris, a prominent jewelry designer, who has been involved with the
university's archaeological project in Peru. Robert visited the excava-
tion site and designed several pieces of jewelry based upon 1,000-year-
old artifacts and architectural detail of the ruins. He plans to donate

the profits from the sale of the archaeology-inspired jewelry to the university—a very generous offer.

I am staying in a fifty-dollar-a-day room at the University Club on Fifth Avenue and 54th Street, a grand old building. Darkly rich, carved panels surround the reading room and reach toward an elaborately-gilded ceiling. Massive tables hold newspapers and magazines being looked over by a couple of elderly gentlemen. On the walls hang a Gilbert Stewart painting of George Washington and several nineteenth-century portraits. My favorite area is the fourth-floor library, where two high walls of books encircle desks illuminated by green lamp shades. There, stairs lead to a second-story walkway which weaves in and out of aisles, so that readers have easy access to all the books. When Rebekah stays here, she traces the circumference of the library rooms on the walkway and pulls dusty books from the deepest shelves. My bedroom is on a level with old books lining the hallways, so when I get off the elevator to go to my room, I feel I am being carried to a time when businessmen sat by the fireplace smoking cigars, reading *The Wall Street Journal,* and women wore thick stacked heels and hats with brims that touched their cheeks. I can almost see these women waiting politely in the Ladies' Lounge for their partners to check long, wool topcoats and white scarfs.

When I left the University Club for Robert's office, rain was pouring and by the time I arrived, my shoes were soaked and feet had turned blue from shoe polish. There I met other university benefactors for a tour of Robert's studio and his shop, followed by dinner at a Japanese restaurant that served very exotic food which everyone had trouble getting into their mouths with chopsticks.

I enjoy coming to New York once in awhile by myself. It holds many memories for me which sometimes seem to come back more easily when I am here alone. Since my surgery, I like having private time just to remember and to think about the course that my life has taken. Early in our marriage, I worked as the Registrar of the American Express Language School—one block away from where I am staying tonight. My former University of Utah sorority sister, Christina Gates, also worked in the office, and together we explored the midtown Manhattan shops, museums, and restaurants. Our husbands were in graduate school, so our budgets were lean compared to our enthusiasm and curiosity. Now I notice that many of the restaurants and shops remain from twenty years ago. My favorite, "La Fondue," located on 55th Street between Fifth and

Sixth Avenues, is still popular as ever, and the fondue and salad taste exactly the same, it seems, as in 1968. The decor has not changed: Orange and olive-green fondue pots—which were a favorite wedding gift in the 1960s—sit on a long, high shelf that surrounds the dining room. Back then I would often walk Sixth Avenue heading toward South Central Park, usually noticing an enormous man draped in heavy fabric and who wore some kind of Nordic head gear. He was known as "The Viking" and stood on the same street corner every day shouting to pedestrians, about what I cannot recall. After passing the Viking, I sometimes would stop at the local grocery store to buy yogurt for lunch, but other times I would use lunch hours to visit the Museum of Modern Art or American Craft Museum. And occasionally I would climb the stairs of Rockefeller Center to give myself a bit of a workout.

When I visit New York, I often feel I am coming home. I have wondered why this is so and think it is because I "grew up" psychologically while living here. When Gordon and I left Salt Lake City—two weeks after our marriage—so that Gordon could attend Columbia Law School, we were both naive—not only about education, but social, political, and cultural issues as well. Everyone we met in New York City seemed articulate, informed, and urbane. One day while browsing through a fabric store by Macy's, two sales clerks commenced a heated argument about the relative merits of presidential candidates Humphrey and Nixon. The arguments of the two clerks were analytical and persuasive, and I left the store feeling absolutely stupid. Many things happened while living in New York that gave voice to deep aesthetic stirrings, but none more than the noon trips to art museums and galleries: Klee's little translucent fish, Renoir's wide Panama hats, Matisse's pink flesh on vivid greens, or Pollock's rich color blendings.

October 4, 1988

While in New York, I saw my friend, Maxine Greene, a philosopher at Teachers College and a very distinguished educator. Maxine is a slender, thin-faced woman who looks more like an elegant, splendidly-dressed wife of a European ambassador than a brilliant university professor. We have been good friends for many years. As I recall, my first acquaintance with Maxine was through an article that she wrote some ten years ago in which she discussed the value of education. She said that education is how we introduce the "newcomers" of the world to life and its meanings and that if we love our children, we will open doors to their potential. Then she continued, as though in poetry, naming for the reader misguided programs and the huge open spaces of a child's possibilities that begin to fold in on him or her if neglected. While I was not involved with education, except as a student, I was transformed by this single writing: There was something startling in the voice behind the words, an insight, a magical light reaching under my skin.

I finally met Maxine when she spoke at West Virginia University seven or eight years ago. Afterward, I wrote to her and sent one of Rebekah's drawings. We corresponded periodically and would occasionally get together when I was in New York. Our friendship continues to grow. We both have had cancer. Mine came first, then recently she developed colon cancer. Gratefully, she now seems fine.

Last April, Maxine stayed at our house in Boulder while she was involved in a university program. It was the day that I was to begin my radiation treatment. The evening prior she had put in very long hours speaking and socializing, and I was concerned about her having jet lag or not getting enough rest. I was prepared to travel alone to Denver for the radiation treatment early in the morning and for someone else to take her to Denver later in the day where she was supposed to give another major address. After I readied myself for the trip, I stopped by Maxine's room to say goodbye. There she stood, already dressed, and quickly announced that she was coming with me, so I would not be alone. Maxine's daughter, Linda, died of breast cancer two years ago, and it was Linda's birthday just the day before. We drove to Denver, and she pretended she was not thinking of Linda. And yet, in the waiting room, I could tell that memories were closing in on her, but she sat poised and spoke to me in a comforting voice.

October 10, 1988

I am working in Boulder today, trying to prepare for my Indiana trip which is quickly approaching. The paper that I will present on the

Ethics of Professional Volunteerism was sent to the symposium participants in advance, so at least I am not rushing to finish it at the last
minute. Today I also must draft a few letters of inquiry to send to
foundations that might be interested in funding the Center's projects.
With the Indiana paper behind me, I might even start writing a grant
proposal to support my new research on gender difference in ethical
decision making by doctors and lawyers. It will be a busy day, but
before starting I will buy a cookie, go for a ride, hopefully engage in
a bit of reflection, and then return to the university in time to attend a
lecture on *The Marriage of Figaro.*

October 17, 1988

I can tell Gordon is stressed, more so than since my surgeries a year
ago. For as long as I have known him, he has always been able to handle
professional pressures remarkably well, almost in a way that seems
unnatural for most people. While he does not talk too much about the
loss of his father, I know it weighs on him and his work. And too,
there are significant issues facing the university right now, such as the
impending privatization of University Hospital and the restructuring
of the Denver-based campus.

Particularly troubling is the tax referendum which, if passed, would
severely limit state funding of higher education and would do irrepara-
ble damage to the university. Unfortunately, the polls show that sixty
percent of the public is behind this measure. Two years ago this same
amendment appeared on the ballot, and Gordon had to work night
and day to beat it then. Now he is putting in an enormous amount of
time, comes home, joins in a quick family dinner, then goes upstairs to
make telephone calls. Somehow I feel that he is distancing himself
from Rebekah and me: There are no quick trips to Dairy Queen,
fewer questions about homework, less back-and-forth teasing and
taunting between Gordon and Rebekah. I ask what is wrong, but
nothing comes back except a few pleasantries. I suggest we go for a
walk, and we do, following single file along the narrow dirt path in the
field where tiny crickets jump through our legs and into the grass until
we meet the bike road where we are able to walk side by side. I ask

Gordon questions, but it seems I am forcing them: "What is bothering you? Why am I always the one who puts the issues on the table? You don't even try to be a part of the family. You just come home and go upstairs. Is something going on at work?" I keep walking, thinking how strange it is to be married to someone for twenty years and yet to feel uncomfortable sometimes posing intimate questions. We start talking, and my self-conscious uneasiness falls away. Finally, Gordon tells me about the pressures, and I think how lonely his world must often be, how infrequently someone ever says "thank you," how he has few friends who can share up and down times. He looks so tired sometimes.

October 18, 1988

I wonder how much longer we can endure this lifestyle. Yes, there are clear advantages to the way we live, but the emotional costs are sometimes high. Often I feel that I am compromising my health. I have difficulty finding walking time, don't take time to eat properly, and am not sleeping well. Never can I use weekends to recover because they are sometimes as busy as the week, with various social functions of one kind or another, correspondence I must answer, or professional deadlines that must be met. For the last few years, Gordon has been gone so much that I doubt we have had more than a single twenty-minute conversation. Then my own professional and university work takes about ten to twelve hours every day, with the remaining waking hours devoted to Rebekah and her care. If I did not have to handle family matters alone, it would not be so hard, but university constraints remove Gordon from much of family life, at least from its daily routines and rhythms. He is away so much in the evening that when he is home it is hard to plug him into Rebekah's homework, piano, social, and sports schedule. She and I are used to going it alone, so even when he is home, Rebekah and I work through our routine and leave Gordon sitting by himself in the family room staring at the television. Sometimes I joke that being a university president's wife is like being divorced, a mother, and holding two full-time jobs. It is supposed to be funny, but it's true.

Gordon does spend time with Rebekah in the morning, gets her up, fixes breakfast, drives her to school, which gives me some quiet time for getting ready and off to work. Many years ago we established this pattern at the suggestion of a woman who was a young child when her father was Governor of West Virginia. She said that her father always set aside early mornings as family time, and that the children knew they could count on this daily availability and attention. Thankfully, a similar arrangement helps our situation and lends some sense of balance in our lives.

October 24, 1988

I just returned from the Indianapolis Conference. Gratefully, my presentation seemed to go well. Justice John Noonan, who sits on the Ninth Circuit Court of Appeals, gave the keynote address. I was one of four presenters whose papers were reviewed by about fifty symposium participants. Since the papers were circulated in advance, the format called for comment and critique rather than a redundant presentation of the paper itself. Most of the symposium members were scholars of religious studies and history, and I felt a bit out of place. Still they were a lively, intelligent group, and I came away excited about the chance to meet some very dynamic scholars and to think about my own research interests from the perspective of religion.

October 28, 1988

Tonight is the school Halloween dance. Rebekah's friend, Lisa, will be coming to our house after school and they may or may not go to the dance—they don't sound terribly enthusiastic about it. If they go, Rebekah will wear an Egyptian costume, a repeat Halloween outfit and Rebekah's favorite.

For a few days, we have had a new residence manager by the name of Kelly Larson. She is the kind of person you want to know, and a very competent individual. She and Rebekah seem to be getting along well.

Having her in our home has reduced the stress that we have been conditioned to feel regarding some staff. She seems excited, involved, never complains, and is having a good effect on us all.

October 31, 1988

Today I am outlining a project to bring in indepth legislative analysis of health care issues. The Colorado legislature, like most state assemblies, has a very small professional staff which really lacks the resources and expertise to undertake thorough analysis of today's complex health care issues. This project would provide a systematic method of identifying and analyzing priority health issues for legislative consideration each legislative term.

Gordon and I went out for breakfast this morning. It gave us a restored sense of communication and warmth to talk for a few minutes. He still is having a rough time with the personal challenges that he has faced this past year with my cancer and his father's death. Normally, Gordon is a very enthusiastic and positive person who has experienced no health, financial, or personal trials of a serious nature. No major calamity or predicament has occurred in his life to test his physical and emotional stamina or challenge his spiritual moorings. He always has been professionally successful, always on top of things, always out there in front, leading the charge. Then within twelve months these two events occur. He has to face separation and loss and recognize for the first time his own vulnerability and mortality. Part of him wants to deny that this is happening, that his father is gone, that I might die. Mostly he keeps the facade in place, the persona of the university president who is "in control," but there are times when I see into him and feel a fragile fear. One day, for example, we were arguing about my attending some social function with him. I felt that I was too busy, and he was pressuring me to accompany him. Finally, he conceded to my view and with a low voice said, "I just want to be with you."

I go to see Dr. Robinson again tomorrow. I found another small lump in my left breast. It is very small, and I am not as nervous about it as I was about the last one.

November 1, 1988

I have returned from my appointment with Dr. Robinson: He feels very confident that this small lesion is of no consequence. Great! Now I am sitting in my home study looking out of the window and thinking that the weather is starting to turn cold. Threatening clouds loom over the mountains. I watch a gray finch struggle to keep its perch on a mostly bare tree branch, its back facing the powerful wind. Tiny feathers on its head stand on end while rain starts blowing hard against the windows, making a grating sound. Details of stone fade from the Flatirons, and a few new gray clouds spread open, revealing blue and white forms that float against the sky—clouds, flocks of birds, stars. There aren't too many more warm days left to walk outside. Soon it will snow, and the path through the field will turn to mud and ice.

November 7, 1988

Today I got up early to take my morning walk in the Crossroads Mall. Now, returned, from the bedroom window I see a few brave souls jogging along the bike path bordering the western boundary of the field, looking cold and attentive to their footing.

I take a shower and wash my hair, noting that it no longer comes out in my hands or falls to the floor and clings to my wet feet. It used to be that I would lift my head in the morning and leave the pillow covered with hair. During chemotherapy, hair was everywhere: on clothing, carpeting, towels, upholstery, bedding, books. Now it is coming back, even a little curly, it seems. The part has filled in, and although my hair still seems thin, I decide to store the hairpiece in a drawer with old hair dryers and curling irons. While my hair lacks shine and a healthy appearance, it continues to improve. Also people are saying my skin color is better, once a former greenish-gray and now pinkish. Finally there are days when I almost forget the cancer, when there are no trips to Denver for radiation or chemotherapy, no pressure in my chest, no red scars, wigs, green skin, fatigue, or nightmares. And yet a thought of death still comes to me when I am going to sleep, and often when I first wake up. Still, I welcome the gift of each day and its new chance to be alive.

November 10, 1988

Tonight was the first evening performance of Rebekah's school play, *Behind the Door*. It is about two elderly matrons who continually talk about their younger sister, who mysteriously remains on the other side of a locked door. Eventually, the ladies convince an unsuspecting stranger to marry their younger sister, sight unseen. At the play's end, the mystery door is opened for the groom, and the young bride, a lifeless corpse, stands on the threshold with hair streaming over a face covered with oatmeal paste. Rebekah was one of the elderly sisters. To achieve the proper effect, she fastened her hair in a bun covered with baby powder to appear gray and wore padding here and there to give a matronly shape. Rebekah had an excellent old-lady shuffle and way of talking, but my favorite scene was the one in which she sat in a rocking chair, knitting and puckering her mouth to seem as though dentures were about to fall out.

Mother and Frank, my stepfather, flew from Salt Lake City to see the performance. They said it was important to experience choice moments with their grandchildren before life passes. I can tell Rebekah is very grateful for caring grandparents who would make such a journey to see her school play.

November 14, 1988

I walked in the mall again this morning. My ghost will haunt this mall, as I haunt it now. My thoughts are different here compared to the field where I am surrounded by songs of the meadowlark, dragonflies darting, periwinkle bells hanging from long slender stems, aromas from damp vegetation, by the beauty of the great mystery—as the Indians say.

Inside the mall, as I walk through partially-lit halls past dark store windows, an inward discourse starts. I think through the schedule of the day: telephone calls; plans for Rebekah; dinner menu; what I forgot to tell Gordon about the weekend; whether I should devote more time to research; how to deal with a difficult employee; if I can lose a few pounds. Often I think about my religion, how it helps me, aspects I like and don't like, and what my theology should tell me in terms of this day. I do get frustrated by what I perceive as its lack of sensitivity to women's concerns—but then I come back to its basic goodness and truth and the spiritual tranquility that constantly answers my fears.

November 22, 1988

Rebekah is prospering with her new piano teacher, Christine Armstrong. She is learning Christmas carols and reviewing old ones, some of which are duets. Though I am not much of a pianist nowadays, I love playing Christmas music with her. The grand piano is in the gallery, which professional musicians say is a very "live" room—sound carries loud and clear. We sit on the piano bench, hips touching, heads beating out the rhythm while she plays the melody, and I work on the accompaniment. "Oh Tannenbaum," is a favorite, along with "Hark the Herald Angels Sing," "Jingle Bells," and "Silent Night." Sometimes we sing and play, and other times just play. If Gordon is home, he often joins in, although usually from a distance. Curiously, he can remember names of people he briefly met five years ago, footnotes to law cases, insignificant battles of the American Civil War, but not the words to songs. His contribution to our recital is, therefore, qualified, but we are grateful for a tenor note here and there.

I can tell Rebekah finds playing the piano relaxing, as I did for the many years I studied piano. Sometimes I walk from the gallery to the back patio where I can hear her and see the field and mountains at the same time.

December 3, 1988

I go back and forth in my feelings about my health and about life and death. Today I feel peaceful, a settling sense of being in the world.

December 10, 1988

It appears we will have a busy social schedule during the holidays. Several parties are planned for our home, including the traditional staff parties, dinner for the University Regents, a reception for Rhodes Scholar finalists, and a party for potential donors to the university.

The edges of our roof are lined with clear white lights, and the large blue spruce by the back yard fountain is covered with red, blue, orange, and green bulbs. Next to the pine is a wooden Santa and sleigh, pulled by four buffaloes, representing the university mascot. Because the turnpike between Boulder and Denver passes our home, Santa, the lights, and even our two inside Christmas trees are visible to motorists traveling this route. Tonight a cold front is blowing in, and the light bulbs are clattering fiercely against the tile roof.

Inside, a large Christmas tree stands in front of the French doors of the gallery and faces the back yard and field. It is decorated simply with white flocking, small white lights, and a few long, crystal icicles. Our family tree, which we are just starting to decorate, is far from simple and soon will be covered with trimmings acquired over many years. Rebekah has selected most of them, so they represent her preferences at various life stages: painted wooden figures and sleighs one year, the next season a few unicorns and dolls, and another time angels with porcelain faces. Two or three Christmases ago, Carolyn, my stepsister, made delicate, starched crocheted stars, and Mother sewed needlepoint squares, with a wreath, gingerbread man, and Santa designs.

This year, we purchased a few Victorian glass ornaments which brought memories of decorating the tree at Grandma and Grandpa Cannon's home. There, trimming the tree was always a family affair. Grandpa would bring the ornaments from the basement and carefully remove them from boxes with small partitions of cardboard. Each ornament was unique and reflected the large primary-colored lights on the tree like fabulous jewels: a red, green, and gold Santa sliding down a chimney, a long, silver and blue pine cone, a pink clear glass ball with white snow crystals dripping down its sides, a gold angel with silver wings. Grandpa would hand my brother and me flat metallic forms, layers of shimmering color which we separated and positioned until creating full, three-dimensional snowflakes in greens, reds, and golds. Grandma placed the Hummel carolers on the marble mantle, donning protective gloves to safely arrange spun glass in folds at their feet; then we built a miniature village on the floor by the tree, illuminated by large white Christmas lights placed through holes in the back of each small structure. My favorite decoration was a small porcelain tree with multicolored bubble lights, slender beakers of liquid that would bubble when heated. Set on a small table, the tree could be seen from the street, glowing through translucent white fabric that covered the glass of the door. After the tree-trimming fuss, the evening would draw in around sounds of quiet laughter and smells of thick chowder and toast. Why mention all of these things? I am not trying to be impressive in my memory of detail, rather I see, in retrospect, the child in myself and where life and my fears have taken me since those delightful and sure times.

December 20, 1988

It is six o'clock in the morning. I am writing in my journal before I dress because I feel the need to preserve certain feelings of the last two days before they go away. I have been tossing and turning in bed for the past couple of nights, unable to sleep. Every night when I turn off the lights, I start wondering how dying will be. Will the dark just close in? Will I feel loved ones slip away? Will I be suffering and welcome relief? Will I be frightened or peaceful? It seems Freud was right: It is impossible to comprehend your own death. I think of my father dying in a horrible airplane accident. What was it like? What was the experience of Gordon's father? What are they feeling now? Something splendid? Or simply nothing? At night, in the dark, I think about being told my cancer has returned. Have the doctors gotten it all? Or, in a few years, will it kill me?

December 22, 1988

I watched a television documentary tonight on experimental cancer treatments. Rebekah is staying at a friend's house, and Gordon is on a trip. Although I usually don't watch much television, I just flipped it on while getting a snack. Several cancer patients were interviewed, including a young redhead in her twenties, a middle-aged man, and another woman probably in her early thirties. The youngest woman and the man died before the documentary was completed. The surviving woman, a victim of stomach cancer, was asked a number of times about her treatment and prognosis. When the camera switched to a reception room, hair rose on my neck. She sat there, lips quivering, eyelids flickering, waiting for doctors to say if her cancer had grown or regressed.

December 23, 1988

In three days Rebekah and I leave for a theater tour of London. This is the first holiday in seven years that I have not gone to a college football bowl game right after Christmas. Gordon will be traveling to California where the University team will play in the Freedom Bowl, and then to Florida for the Orange Bowl. I am looking forward to my London trip, as it will be time to spend with Rebekah. She is a marvelous companion, and I will enjoy some concentrated moments with her. Often Rebekah is so occupied with school, sports, and friends that sometimes I feel we are not connecting as well as we could.

Today, however, Gordon, Rebekah, and I are having some strong family experiences. We are doing a lot of family cooking: sugar cookies, cakes, corn bread, stir-fry chicken. Rebekah loves to combine ingredients, although sometimes she does not heed where or how it should be done. For instance, yesterday she stood in the middle of the family room and ladled flour into a mixing bowl. Gordon never has liked to cook, but he tries to be a good sport, helping to load the dishwasher and sampling hot gingerbread men. Tomorrow, we will do some last minute Christmas shopping: pumpkin and mince pies for dinner, onions and celery for the stuffing, and a few items to put in Christmas stockings.

On top of these holiday preparations, Rebekah and I are trying to pack for Europe, and the Ping-Pong table is stacked with hair dryers, adapters, cassette players, toiletries. No matter how complete our advance preparations, I likely will be up until three A.M. ironing, counting socks, and putting shampoo bottles in plastic bags.

December 25, 1988

This may be my favorite Christmas Day yet, even better perhaps than the year Santa brought loads of new dresses for my Madame Alexander and Muffie dolls. Christmas has fallen on Sunday, so we attended church for a musical program arranged by our friend, Sharon Gerdy. I was asked to be one of the narrators who read part of the Christmas story from the New Testament, so I took my place on the stand and looked at faces in the congregation: two young girls in black velvet dresses with lace collars, a four-year-old boy with red bow tie and slicked-down hair, a grandmother starting to reach under the bench for a squirming toddler, a mother wearing a Christmas corsage with tiny silver bells. Immediately, my stomach filled with butterflies—I get so nervous speaking in church. Gordon is the same way. For all the public addresses he gives, he nearly falls apart when asked to speak in church meetings. Perhaps it is just that we don't have a lot of practice in this setting, but I also know that speaking where the spirit is so present arouses a very reverent and humbling sort of fear. I also worry that I will cry when I speak about my faith, and I usually do.

The music and speakers begin. Words go by, phrases, chords. I do my part and sit down. I look at Gordon and Rebekah. He has his arm around her shoulder. She has tucked her head against his neck. I think about Christ as a child, and I remember when I sat by a Christmas tree and was cradling a three-week old infant while neighborhood carolers sang "Silent Night."

December 28, 1988

London. Rebekah and I are loving this city. We arrived yesterday about 11:00 A.M. Although Rebekah could not sleep on the airplane, she totally collapsed as soon as we arrived at the Russel Hotel. While she rested, I walked around the area, where we are staying, to stretch my legs and get a feel for the neighborhood. London is so very compact that in less than two hours I had found the British Museum, the Theatre District, Regent Street, and Bedford Square—where Virginia Woolf used to meet with the Bloomsbury group.

Today we journeyed to Windsor Castle and Hampton Court, but I totally embarrassed Rebekah on our way. Although I have been to London before, I have never visited the castle so did not know quite what to look for. I was trying to follow the bus map which indicated we were getting close. As we approached a large structure, which I assumed was a building on the castle grounds, I signaled the bus to stop and told Rebekah it was time to get off. We climbed down but then noticed there was no one else around. Seeing our confusion, the bus driver kindly asked, "Where do you want to go?" "Windsor Castle," I replied. At this the other passengers broke into loud laughter. "This is a college," the driver said. "Windsor Castle is still up the road a bit." Sheepishly, we climbed back into our seats, where Rebekah chastised me all the way to the proper stop.

After touring the castle, we had tea in a small confectionery. Just in case peppermint tea and honey are not available, we carry a small supply—Rebekah does not like strawberry jam. We ordered the full traditional tea, with finger sandwiches, pastries, and scones. Rebekah took the cucumber and ham sandwiches which left me the salmon and chicken salad. Both of us saved room for the scones, and Rebekah secretly removed most of the raisins from hers. When the family was in

London last summer, we started to love tea time. And now the white china, the tea, the lemon tarts with candied violets, the chocolate morsel, hands twisting a paper napkin, and some quiet talk continue to be enough pleasure to last for years.

January 5, 1989

Rebekah and I visited Westminster Abbey this morning. Next to having tea, this is my favorite thing to do in London. We arrived early, hoping to miss the crowds, but the cathedral was filled with tourists sitting on chairs, following tour guides, and stooping to read inscriptions. The hum of low-speaking voices echoed around the great dark place.

Slowly we walked through the choir and apse, passed tombs of English nobility and heroes. But after awhile, Rebekah became impatient with my stopping at every marker and soon broke away to explore on her own. For several minutes, I searched for her until we finally met and argued about her running off and rules about travel. My solution was to take her to the brass-rubbing shop located in the crypt and let her copy a brass plate while I saw more. This arrangement worked, and by noon we were both ready to venture onward to shopping and an elegant high tea at Harrods.

We returned to the hotel just in time to dress for the ballet and join University of Colorado theater and music professors Dick Knaub and Dennis Jackson, who came to England also and who serve as our guides. Then we walked to the underground where in just two stops we were in front of the theater where we would see *Giselle*. The building was small and cramped, and our seats were high and close to the stage. Unfortunately, Rebekah forgot her glasses and was frustrated at not being able to see clearly. She and I are at a point where I do not consider myself responsible for remembering everything for her. But she has enjoyed this luxury and resents its absence. The resulting quarrels occur, and now more intensely on this trip when we are locked together in a small hotel room. But we also are experiencing some lovely, intimate moments when our thoughts are compatible and flow harmoniously together.

January 7, 1989

Today was not quite as successful as previous days. We spent almost two hours trying to locate Charles Dickens' home and, when we finally did, found it closed. I have just completed several Dickens' novels, and Rebekah is in the middle of _Great Expectations_, so we were both looking forward to a tour through the author's residence. Initially we took the underground, and then tried walking, following a map. When at last it was apparent that we were off the mark, we hailed a cab which took us right to the spot. Two disappointed-looking people were standing by the front step, reading an oval-shaped plaque and a sign that said "Closed for the season." Then we took our turn staring in the window and door. Actually, we were quite a distance from the main streets and from any underground stop, so not until after walking several blocks could we get a cab to take us to the Victoria and Albert Museum. There we had a light lunch in the museum's rooftop cafe and soon felt sufficiently strengthened to spend several hours studying ornate medieval altarpieces and blue-gold porcelain urns. After we were saturated with museum artifacts, we headed toward Regent Street to take a look at the Christmas decorations which were very different from the plastic, glitzy, color-coordinated trimmings found at home. Rebekah and I decided that their Christmas ornaments are "Victorian," with their dark golds, greens, and red foil garlands. Suspended over Regent Street are decorations unlike anything found on an American main street: Enormous chandelier-styled light fixtures hang from thick cables attached to the tops of buildings. During the day, light filters through the gold, blue, and white glass, and at night they are lit with candle-type lights that sputter and spark, shooting out bright flashes. As Rebekah and I walked arm in arm, I couldn't help thinking, "This life and its simple materiality holds something universally immaterial which lets me see my other face—my inner being."

January 11, 1989

Yesterday we returned from London, and today Rebekah tried very hard to go to school in the afternoon, but she was so exhausted that I doubt she processed anything at all. Unfortunately, her finals begin in less than a week, which means that right away she needs to make up missed work and start reviewing. Of course, we had to stay up for a while to regale Gordon with stories of our adventures, favorite plays, and shopping finds.

Returning to my journal today, I see that I have a hard time writing while on a trip. There are too many distractions, as well as a different kind of daily regimen. My journal hardly mentions any of the twelve or thirteen performances we saw on our tour—when the principal reason I took Rebekah is that she enjoys theater, in particular Shakespeare. We saw musicals, drama, ballet, and a Christmas "Panto" or pantomime. Rebekah was less taken with *Phantom of the Opera* than with Tennessee Williams' more serious *Orpheus Descending*. Initially, I was worried that some of the performances planned for the trip might be too heavy, sexual, or violent for an almost thirteen-year old but she seemed to get a lot out of almost everything we saw. Our guides, Dick and Dennis, took care to explain Williams' treatment of women and the long history of the British "Panto" tradition. When we took a side excursion to Stratford-upon-Avon, the Shakespeare Memorial Company was performing the Plantagenet Series consisting of three historical plays. I thought Rebekah would not like to sit through more than one, so I made alternative arrangements to see a romantic farce performed in the tradition of Restoration Theater. She did not like the Restoration play at all and complained throughout the evening that we did not have more tickets to Shakespeare. With a bit of negotiating, I was able to secure tickets to *Richard III* and *Henry IV, Part I*. We attended both, and she was absolutely enthralled with the drama and action. Off and on for the rest of the trip, she mimicked Richard III by stuffing her sweater under the shoulder of her coat and walking with a great sideways-dipping limp.

January 12, 1989

Ever since returning to Colorado, I have felt drawn to the field, so about four o'clock this afternoon I decided to try cross-country skiing on the open grounds behind the house. The sun is shining, and the glare of the snow is so bright that even with dark glasses I have to squint. Snow fell yesterday evening but now in the afternoon, it looks almost toasted on top by the blazing sun. It is sufficiently deep that I can take a few awkward steps over the gardens and be perfectly positioned in the smooth, snow-covered field. I have not attempted this sport for several years, so I cautiously take the first sliding steps through the white. The first stroke, the skis glide on the surface. Then they abruptly break through the crust as my body weight shifts. Unless I lift the toe of the ski before placing it, it slides under the snow's hard surface and disappears. After several comedic attempts to coordinate swings of arms and legs, I glide to the very middle of the field, an area where I seldom walk because in other seasons the grass is high and rough. Now the field is glossy and sleek, and a slight wind swirls lifting ice crystals for sunlight to snatch. Then reversing my course, I circle past an old, tall cottonwood tree where a few winter finches spring from branch to branch, fluttering up a few feet then alighting almost exactly where they set off.

🙩 *"The Readiness Is All"*

January 22, 1989

Today I had my fifth chemotherapy treatment. Once again I saw my oncologist, Dr. Robinson—an internationally recognized cancer specialist but also a competent, caring, and humble human being. Throughout these past months, I have always felt that he respects my need to understand my cancer. This morning we discussed a few research and journal articles or news stories I had read and their relevance to my case. Occasionally, we consider new diagnostic tests for breast cancer; other days, I have suggested tests or procedures, such as a bone-density test or bone-scan evaluation, and Dr. Robinson attentively listens, sometimes agreeing with my assessment. He believes patients do better if they play an active role in their care and treatment instead of being passively involved. Never once have I felt that he regarded me as an "object," a complaint often leveled against physicians. And after an examination or treatment session, he puts his arms around my shoulders and pulls me toward him in an almost fatherly way. Recently, a nurse told me that Dr. Robinson drives about fourteen hours per month between Aspen and Denver to conduct breast clinics, and that on Christmas Day, he serves dinner at the homeless shelter. I know that he regularly works holidays at the hospital, so that residents can have the day with their families. Many times, I have wondered if he realizes the effects of his caring manner, but if asked, he would probably respond that he is just doing his job.

On the way home from treatment, I thought about Dr. Robinson and the other people who consistently treat and care for me. No doubt, I feel a strong dependency because in important respects they are more in control of my life than am I. My understanding of how my body works is very limited and almost juvenile; but while I ought to know more about T-cells and estrogen and ways they relate to my cancer, I don't have time for indepth study. In a way, I am afraid to know more than I do, so I have to give over part of myself to someone else and live with this unsettling, almost helpless feeling; yet there is more than the dynamics of dependency that infuses how I see these doctors and nurses. Maybe it's because we take time to share stories about children, work schedules and vacations that I feel a growing and personal attachment.

Sometimes I think it must be more difficult for doctors and nurses to understand their feelings toward patients because they must watch not to become so personally involved that they can't help. Still, it would be hard to see a young man every day for months, visit with his family, cradle his child and not despair when his lungs fill with fluid, and he dies. I think that this is the vulnerability I sense in Dr. Robinson.

January 25, 1989

I saw Dr. Robinson today for a routine examination. For a while, we conversed about his melanoma research and some promising findings, and then we spoke generally about what we both had been doing since I last saw him. I asked about recent news stories indicating that Beth Israel Hospital in Boston had developed an experimental blood test that could be used to detect the presence of cancer. He was monitoring the research and even requesting some blood samples to see how reliable the test is. We talked about possibly getting involved in experimental trials, but concluded it would be best to wait until more data was available.

On the way home, I thought about the difference between how I felt on this trip to see Dr. Robinson and those I took almost a year ago when I was starting radiation treatments. Although I don't think I will ever forget the terror, anger, and humiliation of those days—and it is probably best that I don't forget—the feeling of indignation is gone, along with the denial and hurt. Rarely does a day pass that I do not think of the cancer, wondering if it will return, but the thought does not come alone now. Instead, it is accompanied by a vision of geese against the pale purple sky, weeds dividing the snow drifts, and Rebekah's piano chords floating out onto the field at dusk.

These days, I think more about the theology of my religion, what it says about birth, death, immortality, and divinity, and I see more and more how it fits with other psychological and philosophical frameworks—even physics. Right now I am reading a few works by Joseph Campbell, and am struck, as was he, by the repeating themes that underlie mythological symbols and metaphors, how ideas go different ways to the same end, toward a suggestion of awakening, a turning both inward and outward at the same time to what Campbell calls "the horrendous power that is of all creation." I don't think my beliefs are a mere coping mechanism, but rather a gift of truth in which I am enlightened by a wondrous story about what it means to be human.

February 1, 1989

Rebekah missed school this morning to attend part of a conference on global warming held at the law school. Gordon picked her up, and the three of us met at the university. For a long time, she has been very interested in this issue and has studied it some in school. The conference honored Nick Doman, our good friend, who with his wife, Kitsy, has rendered strong support of the university and the law school. During the program we sat next to Kitsy and listened to excellent presentations that raised profound concerns about the causes and solutions to a very real threat.

We see the Domans every once in awhile, either in New York or when they come to Colorado. They are both intelligent, well-traveled, and full of stories about harrowing excursions to Eastern Block countries. Nick was one of the prosecuting attorneys at the Nuremberg Trials, and as a result of his expertise in international law was invited to be an observer at the trial of Klaus Barbie who was being tried for his Nazi "crimes against humanity" in Lyon, France—the same charge made at Nuremberg. Now in Boulder, we also talked about the strength of the prosecutor's case, the credibility of Barbie, and the ability of witnesses to identify him after more than forty years. I always enjoy conversations with Nick and Kitsy and go away feeling as though I have just heard a graduate lecture in international law.

February 3, 1989

Gordon and I are attending a meeting of the Business Higher Education Forum in Scottsdale, Arizona, a collaborative effort by select CEOs of major United States corporations and university presidents. It is a distinguished group that wields enough collective power that they should accomplish anything they set out to do. I attend some of the meetings but also relax a bit on the deck overlooking the Arizona valley, letting the sun warm me. February is a great time to come on a trip such as this: Colorado is usually in the thick of weather and snow, while here the saguaro cacti reach out like hands trying to touch the bright sun that swells over rounded, red-brown hills. I order fresh strawberries for breakfast and sit outside, then later with Gordon join some other presidents of large public universities for lunch. Once in awhile, at occasions such as this, Gordon and I are able to meet other couples who are in situations similar to ours, allowing us to share pleasures, frustrations, and challenges with people who understand exactly what we're talking about. Today we discussed the increasing ethnic tension on campuses, but also some of the more humorous moments of public life. Gordon had us nearly hysterical with laughter when he told about how in Florida he was mistaken for the nerdy Burger King "Herb" by a group of screaming teenagers. And I told how four-year-old Rebekah protested leaving her television program when a sitter tried to bring her downstairs to meet The Chief Justice of the United States, Warren Burger. Rebekah stood at the top of the second floor landing and shouted, "The Chief Justice stinks!" A more recent situation involved Caspar Weinberger's visit to the University of Colorado when he was Secretary of Defense. Gordon said he looked out of a window, and saw the Secretary bent over the hood of Gordon's car with the Secret Service wiping something off of the back of his pants. The car had been borrowed to escort Secretary Weinberger to his various campus destinations, and in true military fashion, they put him in the back seat—where Rebekah had been eating a chocolate bar the previous evening.

February 5, 1989

We just returned from our trip. Gordon and I did not leave Arizona until afternoon, so that we could have time for a quiet breakfast together and a walk up the mountain path behind the hotel. We had a good Southwestern-style meal and some much needed quiet talk—about nothing in particular. Assuredly, Gordon and I need to get away once in awhile, to explore the inner territory of marriage that often seems to elude us as a result of the onslaught of the outer public world.

February 13, 1989

Tomorrow Gordon and I meet with the doctors who have been involved with my cancer surgery and treatment: Dr. Byyny, my internist; Dr. Robinson, my oncologist; and Dr. Ketch, my surgeon. Dr. Byyny thought it would be a good idea to review my current status and prognosis. I agree that this meeting is timely, especially in light of the biopsies that I continue to undergo and some rather conflicting reports that I have read recently about survival rates for my stage and type of cancer.

February 14, 1989

I am feeling good about the meeting with my doctors. The more I learn about breast cancer and its treatment, and even my own condition, the more I am able to appreciate the complexity of the disease and the human condition. One of the major issues that we addressed was if I would benefit from further surgery and from removing more breast tissue. Since the last biopsy, when cancer seemed a good possibility, my doctors and I have continued to talk about a simple mastectomy. Dr. Ketch pointed out that there is no good controlled research indicating that breast cancer is reduced by the kind of breast operation I had—a subcutaneous mastectomy—although there are anecdotal reports of benefit. However, the main reason for the lack of evidence is that such a study would be very difficult to conduct and would involve identifying and following women for twenty years who had my particular problem and surgery. Dr. Robinson remarked that I still run the risk of developing a second cancer in the opposite breast at the rate of one percent a year for the rest of my life because what tissue was left is unhealthy. While the chance of cancer developing in the breast that was radiated is very low, the opposite one is a more likely site of a new malignancy, or one that would be unrelated to my previous cancer. In discussing whether a full mastectomy would remove sufficient additional tissue to reduce the likelihood of developing a second cancer, the doctors concluded that the benefit would be slight compared to possible complications of surgery. Dr. Ketch thinks that old scar tissue might mask a problem, and Dr. Byyny believes examination would be harder after such surgery, since ribs and scar tissue might mask a cancer. Now physical examination is fairly easy because implants were placed under the muscle, pushing the breast tissue to the top of a smooth surface. Recalling that he removed ninety-five percent of the breast tissue, Dr. Ketch remarked that a simple mastectomy would result in the elimination of only a bit more because some extending under the arm would have to be left.

All five of us agreed that additional surgery, without evidence of cancer, would not enhance my current situation. That was a relief, because, since my most recent cancer scare, I have been worried about having to undergo another operation. We also talked about the possibility of recurrence, so Dr. Robinson formulated my risk factors: strong family history of cancer, relatively young age, some remaining breast tissue, and an aggressive type of cancer. In my favor was the fact that no evidence of cancer could be found in the dissected lymph nodes and that I had been given both radiation and adjuvant chemotherapy. Dr. Robinson believes the recurrence risk to be small, although chances of developing a second breast cancer are substantially higher. Yet early detection should be easy. I felt reassured when he said that the possibility of dying of cancer was not much greater than dying from other causes. Gordon and I parted from the doctors, feeling that we were on the right track and that the best plan was to continue with regular monitoring and examination. I left the meeting, relieved and very grateful for the competent care I have received, even if the doctors have seemed, at times, to be groping for answers and ideas.

February 21, 1989

I keep thinking about existence, the parts of life: the natural and the man-made, the constructed and the given, the mental and the physical, time and space, mind and soul. When I step onto the deck at night and look at the sky, I wonder what parts of our being cease with death, how we exist in spiritual form, how recognizing the spiritual enhances our grasp of what Mortimer Adler asks, "what man is, how his mind operates, what the soul is, what manner of existence and action (man) would have apart from matter . . . ?"

Daily I think of my father, of Gordon's father, of my grandparents, and especially stories Grandma Cannon told about family, the story of the death of Grandma's younger brother, "Little Heber": Heber died at an early age, about twelve years old. Although I do not recall the nature of his illness, I remember that he had had tuberculosis in his leg. At his death, the family gathered in his bedroom, and my grandmother, a young woman then, remembers that everyone in the room was suddenly aware that Heber's mother, who had died earlier of cancer, was sitting in a nearby empty chair. She had come for her son.

March 1, 1989

Daily life has the illusion of a linear progression because we psychologically experience one occurrence following another, and we reason from premise to conclusion. That is to say, we experience knowledge as cumulative, progressing toward an overall effect. If life is infinite, the word *time* undoubtedly has another meaning.

I try to think not only of an afterlife but also of the pre-life that my religious doctrine describes, where spirit personages had many capacities for learning and progressing into another time framework and came to mortality to gain certain critical knowledge. I wonder what, from that pre-existence, we are able to call upon as help in this dimension. Are we limited in our access to such knowledge by our fixating on a linear experience? Maybe the concepts of time that we take for granted are, in fact, a deception and there are other reasoning capacities and resources for learning.

Even though I normally have a highly-rational orientation to life, many times I have felt a great spiritual understanding. One of the most powerful of these transcendent experiences occurred ten years ago after I had developed an enlarged ovary. It was at the point at which doctors were watching me, telling me that surgery would be necessary if the ovary did not reduce in size within a few weeks. I remember waking to fear every morning, feeling a daily terror. The anguish continued until one day I was attending church, at a time when the congregation was watching a satellite broadcast of one of the church's general conferences in Salt Lake City. The room was dark, so that the screen was clearly visible. The Mormon Tabernacle Choir was singing. Suddenly, I had a rushing feeling of love and understanding, a collage of images: grandparents, family gardens, comforting voices of loved ones, familiar music. The fear was gone. Even to the moment of being wheeled into surgery, it never returned. A friend and nurse stood by my side as I waited on a cot outside the operating room. I told her I had no fear, that I felt a peace about what was happening. Later, she told her colleagues what an extraordinary outlook this was in a patient.

March 10, 1989

My professional work will be demanding this week, so I must be extra careful that it doesn't nudge out my walking and journal writing, or dull the details of the dusty-green sage that I pass on my drive to Denver. Sometimes it is so easy for the soul to start unraveling, snagged by stacks of mail, telephone calls, meetings. This week I am working on a project proposal dealing with gender differences in ethical decision making. Yet, I still need to complete parts of the methodology section and refine the interview protocol. Also, I am revising a proposal to establish a Governor's Task Force on "Life and the Law," which will explore issues of fetal research, organ transplantation, and death and dying.

Then I must think a bit about surveying nurses on the subject of withholding and withdrawing life-sustaining treatment. Finally, I am developing an agenda for a forthcoming meeting in Kansas City to explore a project that would measure the cost-effectiveness of treatments covered by health insurance.

Rebekah tells me today that she transferred out of home economics into computer science because, in her words, "It was so boring." She came home complaining that the home economics teacher had given them a "stupid" test, one requiring written definitions of such terms as *baste, julienne,* and *sauté*. She was absolutely insulted!

March 13, 1989

Today is a voluptuous spring day, the first of the season. This morning I gave myself permission to drive through the countryside for about forty-five minutes. When possible, I love to ride through the farmland that stretches eastward from Boulder where traces of green appear in the brown earth, and the land seems tranquil. The morning sun is high, the sky clear blue and free of clouds. For a few brief moments, I think about being alive, watching the road unfold before me then I feel warm air coming through a crack in the window.

March 17, 1989
(first entry)

I have been reading Grandma Cannon's enlightening journal when working in my law school office. One entry describes the death of her daughter, Florence, from breast cancer. When I glanced through it again today, it evoked many tensions: tensions about ways I wanted to change my life, about the prospect of death, my inadequate faith that there is an afterlife.

This is Grandma's story:

Tuesday, January 17, 1933

After Florence's death, I thought I would like to make a record of those weeks preceding it, yet I have never felt I could stand the heart pull necessary. It is a year now and still it is hard to write about it, but the urge is still upon me . . .

I was busy with my regular house hold tasks. It was about ten in the morning when George (my Grandfather Cannon) came in with a telegram from Dale (Florence's husband). He gave it to me to read, and it said the doctors in Washington had diagnosed her case as a malignant growth, or in other words, a cancer of the breast. Of course the news came as a thunderbolt from the clear sky. . . . A year, the proceeding August, Florence had noticed a small lump in her breast. . . . Florence wrote us about it and we agreed with her that it better be taken out. When the doctor began the operation, he found the growth much deeper than he had expected, and instead of its being just a simple little operation, it was quite an extensive one. The consulting physicians made the examination of the tissues . . . and said it was not a cancerous growth. When we received that news all our fear of that disease was allayed, and I never gave it serious thought there after.

. . . George asked Dale whether Flo was able to travel, and he said he thought she could come home alone. . . . The following morning, George and I were up at six taking the train for Ogden. We arrived in Ogden around seven or eight—I just don't remember the time—there was a wait of an hour or so before the train from the east arrived. It was a beautiful Sabbath morning, a light snow fell the night before, and everything looked so pure and white. . . . When we got to the depot, the children were there and it was a happy reunion for us all. Florence took her father's arm and walked through the station to the car. She said she had not walked that far for over a week. Charlotte (the housekeeper) had a nice dinner ready, and I had tried to have things which I thought she would like. . . . She ate very little, trying, I knew, to do her best. . . . She had a hard time sleeping, and so we talked. It was the only time we talked about her dying. She said how serious her condition was and did I think she might not be going to get well.

. . . The next morning, I helped her wash her hair and take a bath. When I saw her breast and that ugly sore, I felt as the doctor who had seen her last did—that there was the seat of the trouble, and I can never understand how any doctor with average intelligence could see a condition such as that and not think it was serious.

. . . I tried everything I could think of to get Florence to eat. She had no appetite and would only take a mouthful at a time, sometimes going a day without anything. One day after a real trying time, when I had rather urged her to take food, she was so sick, and I said, "Never again will I ask you to eat. I can't stand to see you suffer. I think you know best what you can do." That was nearly a month before her passing, and never did I urge her to take anything. I would prepare food after that day and take it to her, and she ate or not as she wished. . . . It was hard for her to move around every time we gave her a bath: no matter how gently we moved her, it would cause nausea. We would move her from one bed to another and make her bed fresh, but even that much lifting would start the stomach sickness, so for over a month we never tried to move her, only from one side of the bed to the other.

. . . I find this narrative extremely difficult to write, as my eyes are blinded with tears as I write when I review in my mind those anxious days, those sleepless nights. When every waking moment there was a prayer on my lips for her deliverance from these trying hours. What pain can rack the human body before the spirit is finally released? How one does reflect on the various ways death enters. . . . One does not try to understand these various calls of death, but it is just a matter of wonderment. . . . There *are many inexplicable things in life. Life itself is an enigma. Whence comes this spark of life, we say, from another sphere; but then, the wonder is what before that and so on. . . . One thing that I said to myself during those days of pain was "Christ, the perfect man, the man without sin suffered as no human being ever suffered . . . , or at least died a bodily death of exquisite suffering. . . . Why did Mary, the mother of the Christ, have to pass through this ordeal? . . . What were her feelings as she stood at the foot of the cross, helpless, yet willing if it were possible to take his place, and endure what he was called to endure if he might only be spared. A mother, when she sees her offspring suffer, would willingly change places . . . and she could bear the pain again and again for her child's sake. But Mary did stand at the foot of the cross, and undoubtedly called upon her God for help, for strength to witness that death struggle of her beloved son, and God did give her strength, he built up in her an endurance . . ." In this way I talked to myself.*

Florence's sickness was swift and severe: She would have an occasional day when she would feel a little better than the day before, but when I would look back a week, I knew she was much worse than a week before, never was she as well as the first day she arrived, or the second, or third, and so on. . . . She took scarcely any food, just a mouthful now and then; even water she could not swallow. We gave her chopped ice, day and night. She would keep a small piece in her mouth most of the time she was awake. I suppose her calling for ice will ever ring in my ears.

One day when she had been in such pain that she had been moaning and vomiting, she looked at me with a most pleading look and called out, as one would call for succor in a crisis: "Oh mother, don't hold me any longer." That was a month or more before she went. As soon as I could control myself enough to answer, I said, "My darling, I am not holding you. I suffer with you." I think she realized that I did not want to hold her a minute. Day after day I sat by her bed, held my hand on her abdomen because she seemed to think I knew where to put my hand to sooth her. My other hand was on her head or holding it as she reached and vomited. It seemed to me that she vomited thousands of times. She had such severe coughing spells, and that would start the pain in her breast. The ice in her mouth would often prevent her coughing, and sometimes just while I was going into the lavatory to empty some of the vessels, she would feel that she would cough, and then she would call, "Ice!" It seems to me now, often when I am here alone I can hear her call, "Ice!"

I did pray that she could go easily. The doctor did not want to give her too much morphine, and only when her pain was unbearable did they administer it. The last day, he suggested she might take a pill. . . . We persuaded her to try and swallow one. The effort she made to swallow it nearly cost her life. She was unconscious for some time after the effort, and the nurse and we all thought it had killed her. However, she revived and passed a fairly comfortable day. But along towards night, her pulse which had kept up so wonderfully became intermittent, and both nurses thought the end was near.

It came at a little past 11:00 P.M. Very peaceful, and with no struggle. . . . I was thanking my Father in Heaven that she could go so peacefully. Even if I had not had the hope of eternal life, I would have been glad to see her pass. I felt I had reached the limit of human endurance. Anything was preferable to seeing her suffer. Oh, but the glorious thought that she was free from suffering, and that all of it rebounded to her glory; that she had "fought the good fight," that she had kept the faith, and "that she had gone home to that God who gave her life" gave me joy unspeakable. . . . Death melts the heart and makes us all kin in sorrow. . . . George and I felt we would feel better to have her home. George suggested that we all kneel in prayer before we went to our homes and to bed. That prayer is one that will stand out in my memory as long as life lasts. It was one of beautiful resignation, one of comfort and hope. . . . So, in the evening, they brought the body home, and we could see it as long as we liked. I did not sleep that night, and so after all were asleep, I came down and stayed a while and took my last look at her, or at least my last look while I was alone. I reviewed her life in memory: the night she was born, when the doctor said that I was as near gone as one ever gets (I had a severe hemorrhage). I thought how glad Grandma Grant would be to see her, because Grandma only saw her once or twice. . . . I thought how glad my mother would be to see her, and how happy they would all be. I remember what a darling baby she was, so beautiful to look upon that I believed there never had been a more beautiful child. . . . I remember her in early childhood and her happy school days. . . . I thought of her wedding day which had been so happy, and how radiant she was as she went away. I remember my delightful visit with her in Washington, and how I admired her as a woman. . . . Then I thought of how often since her home coming that she had turned to me. How she wanted me by her all the time, and what a comfort it had been to me that I could give her my whole attention. . . . I knelt by the coffin and thanked God for her and said how willingly I gave her up. . . . The experience has been a hallowed one. I am a better woman from having passed through it.

I finished reading and wept hard and deep. Then I dropped to my knees and prayed for peace, asking why it could not be more constant with me. After a few minutes, the stress suddenly lifted, and a contentment circled like a warm current of air.

March 17, 1989
(second entry)

An important challenge of my cancer is to be more "in" life, not to take leave from how I live now, and not to go somewhere and meditate but to bring new dimensions to the life I now have.

March 18, 1989

Last night we had a school party for two groups of students: one was from the Talented and Gifted program at Rebekah's school, the other from the University Student Government. Dinner was a taco bar and other Mexican treats. The students stayed for a long time— eating, visiting, watching television, and playing Ping-Pong. When I walked into the loft to see how the Ping-Pong match was going, one of the junior high boys was squatting at one end of the table, mouth wide open to catch the flying white balls. As the ball came his direction, he would rise and snap and then quickly return to his squatting position.

When Rebekah works at school projects, I sometimes indulge in watching her hands, long fingers that press computer keys, shuffle disordered stacks of wide-ruled paper, or saw dull scissors through colored sheets. All today she labored hard making an origami mobile for her science class. Each suspended object is shaped like a type of crystal. As ever, she exercised great patience throughout the tedium of cutting paper, gluing little flaps in place, decorating with thick paint and glitter, and tying knots in fine thread.

March 21, 1989

On my way home from Denver today, Kelly, our house manager, paged me to say that Rebekah went for a bicycle ride but had not come home on schedule. I sat back in the car, and a tension spread down my neck and across my shoulders. Then I sped along the turnpike to the exit close to our neighborhood. Could I remember what she was wearing this morning? Was she hit by a car? Kidnapped? How long does one wait before calling the police? Just two years ago, a child in Rebekah's school was struck by a slow-traveling car. He almost died and now never will be normal. Looking for a silver-blue bike, I drove around several neighborhood blocks stopping to check houses of people we know. While I drove, I thought what I would do if I found Rebekah: take her bike away, remind her of the family rules? Sometimes she visits her math teacher, Mrs. Bowen, other times the Manteys, Knaubs, or Fronzacks. Not there. I drive further from home, closer to the park, circle a church and pond. Finally, I try the home of Jennifer Eldredge, a schoolmate of Rebekah's. To my relief the bike is propped against a tree, and I see Rebekah visiting with Jennifer on the front porch.

Tonight Rebekah went to "etiquette night" at church. As an act of independence, she was determined not to wear the requisite dress, but she took a skirt with her just in case peer pressure became too strong. When she sat on the stairs pulling on her shoes, I was struck by her beauty and youth. Her blouse of soft blues brought out the gray-blue color of her eyes and many delicate shades of pink in her cheeks, chin, and brow.

March 23, 1989

Gordon returned completely exhausted from a four-day trip to New York. When he walked off of the plane, there was an emergency message waiting at the gate, telling him he had to go to the legislature. He went directly there and, through an extraordinary, sustained effort, succeeded in getting his hospital organization bill to go through. Arriving home late in the evening—about 3:00 A.M. New York time—he could only sit in the chair and gaze straight ahead. How he works such long hours day after day, night after night, I cannot comprehend; even during the day, his work is not like that of most people. "He has to be on stage all day," I always say, meaning that there is no "down" time, that the adrenalin has to be pumping hour after hour—for meetings, for presentations, for speeches. The other day I gave a talk in Denver, and by the time that I drove back to Boulder I was so tired that I could not even write a letter. Giving two or three major addresses in the morning and still being coherent enough to have afternoon meetings is a feat I cannot imagine.

March 26, 1989

Yesterday Rebekah left for Space Camp in Huntsville, Alabama, so Gordon and I have Easter Sunday to ourselves. It has been a quiet Easter. In the morning, we attended church, but have been home all evening. While my intention was to spend time this afternoon writing in my journal, somehow I just couldn't get into it. Already I am feeling tired, defeated that the day got away from me without a single accomplishment. Every once in awhile, it seems I am on a treadmill, going from one insignificant task to the next without making any progress. That is what it has been today: making the bed, straightening the bathroom, putting away dishes, feeding the dogs, sorting mail. It just goes on and on.

Rebekah was very enthusiastic about attending Space Camp because she would like to be an astronaut and particularly would like to go to Mars with the first mission. Her knowledge of the U.S. Space Program is astounding, and I find it both surprising and rewarding to suddenly be in a position in which my child is significantly more informed about some subject than am I—in which I am the learner, and she is the teacher. As Gordon and I waited at the gate for Rebekah's plane to leave, we agreed how independent she has become, how she has developed friendships, made good academic progress, and simply has become a considerate, responsible individual. Then as the plane pulled away, our eyes moistened a little.

As I sit at my desk now, I watch children flying a kite. It is just a little spot against the clouds and blue sky, reminding me of when my father helped my brother and me build a kite. We flew it from our driveway while it was up very high, like this one. Finally, it did not need much help, so when we had to come in for dinner, we tied it to the front sprinkler, and it flew alone.

March 29, 1989

When I took my walk in the mall this morning, I started thinking about womanhood and a few things that I have been reading. Sometimes I think being a woman is the type of existence that Hamlin Garland described when he referred to life on the "Middle Border." Anyone who has flown over the Midwest plains has seen the Middle Border. To Garland, it was a spread of wilderness, a hyphen connecting genteel tradition and frontier adventure. Garland's writing shattered the pastoral romanticism carried in more common sentimental accounts of Midwest farm life. He told what it really meant to be human, on the Middle Border: to be alive here was to be a tragic rider on a perpetual circuit of sameness and oppression. Garland sympathized with the plains' wife. She was the least free, the most hopeless of all, forever turning from one drudgery to the next.

April 1, 1989

It has been close to a year and a half since my cancer surgery. I often think about other women who have breast cancer. Can they put cancer behind them, or is there always something that keeps it near? Constantly, I am struck by how present thoughts of cancer are in my everyday life. "Will I have a recurrence soon?" Will Dr. Robinson detect an enlarged lymph node under my arm or say my cough means that cancer has metastasized to my lungs? Lately, I have felt shooting pains in my forearms, so I imagine it is in my bones.

April 2, 1989

I just returned from a four-day trip to San Francisco where I attended the annual meeting of the American Educational Research Association. Although I was not on the program, I wanted to hear the papers and make some contacts in the Division on Professional Education.

On the plane ride home, I finished reading *Portrait of a Lady*, by Henry James, a book that has been my steady companion since my cancer surgery. For a year and a half, I have taken this book in small doses, savoring just a few pages at a time. If you have cancer, there is much to learn in the story of Isabel Archer. She is an innocent, almost childlike American woman who, during the course of the novel, develops the capacity for critical reflection. As her story unfolds, Isabel transforms an outlook of self-deception to truthfulness and free agency, thus becoming able to critically face her life.

The book begins when she is a young, self-confident, American taken to England by her aunt. There she is determined to have her independence and to control her own life. And yet the problem is that her freedom is proportionate to her imagination and experience; consequently, she misjudges the worth of many characters who try to connect to her in one way or another—as lovers, family, and friends. Isabel thinks that she is free; yet in truth, she is the least free of the men and women in the story: She has imagination, but it is only the inventiveness of fancy and whim, "a tangle of vague outlines," and not an imagination informed by insight, knowledge, and observation.

Isabel finally gives her perception vision, and in so doing sets herself free from the confinement of her marriage. When she finally realizes her husband's intimacy with Madame Merle, a person of preeminent stature in Isabel's mind, imagination meets knowledge, and Isabel begins to truly see. It is then her vision becomes "an active condition: it was not a chill, a stupor, a despair; it was a passion of thought and speculation, of response to every pressure." In so awakening, she became an autonomous moral agent, free to be as she might.

April 3, 1989

Today my reading on gender and law led me to think about some of the women who dwell on "the Middle Border," Isabel Archer, and the meaning of their freedom, especially those who live in the silent spaces of abuse, poverty, oppression, and even cancer. The young abandoned black woman who is on her own to raise four children in a drug-ridden ghetto finds no liberty in her world, no freedom in her choices, no authority in her own language, only convention, prejudice, fate, and the sheer banality of much that defines contemporary culture. Like Thomas Hardy's "Tess," whose life was a tragic story of submission to orthodoxy and fate, the stories of many women become nameless narratives.

April 9, 1989

Sunday. The family stayed home from church because we are all battling illness. I am recovering from a mean cold that did not respond to treatment with antibiotics, and I hope that Rebekah is not getting it. She has a sore throat. Gordon's ears are bothering him.

Lunch was pasta and salad, then Rebekah made a chocolate cake according to her grandmother's recipe—once in awhile we find a dessert recipe that rivals this one, but not very often. After the meal, Gordon loaded the dishwasher, and I put away the food while the dogs that had just been let into the family room chased each other around the chairs, sliding so hard on the slick wood floors that they banged sideways into walls. This weekend Rebekah went to a school party but is being rather secretive about her dancing partners. She said she had to hide out a few times, so that a rather persistent boy would not monopolize her the whole evening. Boys call quite frequently now, and late afternoons mean low murmurs inside her bedroom. Yesterday she received a call from her friend, Daryl, a young man she met at Space Camp who lives in Oahu, and I wondered how dealing with Rebekah and boys will be. Gordon teases Rebekah that he plans to greet her dates at the door in full academic regalia.

Later in the day, Rebekah and I assembled the furnishings for our two doll houses. This has been on my list of things to do for over a year, so it felt good to finally cross it off. The empty pink and blue houses have been sitting upstairs in the family room waiting for us to unpack the furniture. We have gathered dolls, furniture, and other items from our travels and also from cities where we have lived: an antique lace rug from Brussels, a china set from a store adjacent to the "Old Curiosity Shop" in London, a pair of porcelain twin babies from New Orleans. We bought the doll houses when Rebekah was about two years old from a miniature toy store in Provo, Utah. Once she saw the doll houses, she became hysterical. Trying to calm her with, "I just don't think you are ready for a doll house," she loudly replied, "I'm ready for a doll house! I'm ready for a doll house!" until I finally carried her outside through a group of curious onlookers. Of course I thought Rebekah really had to have that doll house for Christmas, just as Gordon, a few years later, would feel that Santa should give her an electric train.

Thinking about the doll houses makes me realize I should include more stories in my journal about Rebekah's early childhood, and even my own, because only a few photo albums, videotapes, and scrapbooks comprise our family history. And too, I am learning that writing about experiences which took place long ago helps me keep my past alive and to remember that my life has been very full, an appreciation that sometimes diminishes as memories fade.

April 10, 1989

I am glad it is Monday. Weekends are always a little disorienting, simply because they are unstructured. Since my surgeries I have tried to maintain a type of program that starts in the morning and continues through the day, providing a constancy that gives me a sense of being in charge of my life. I follow my morning routine to a tee—walk in the mall, take some time for prayer and meditation, study Scriptures, and write in my journal, all by 9:00 A.M.

Tonight Gordon and I are going out for an early dinner. We keep trying to be more regular in this, hoping we might have some time to talk. Often we review our respective schedules for the following couple of weeks, noting when we will be out of town, when we will host social functions, or need someone to stay with Rebekah. I don't care much for this "business" part of our date, however necessary it is; but afterwards we talk about more personal matters: how work is going, when a major university grant is about to be announced, when we might travel together, family time, how Gordon's mother is doing, when Rebekah needs an allergy shot. The death of Gordon's father is still on our minds, and often we reminisce about him or talk about when we might next see Gordon's mother. Gordon seems to be dealing with his loss in a constructive way. Recently, he dictated three tapes about his father, just to record some of his personal feelings and remembrances. While we are together, Gordon and I do not talk about my cancer much anymore because I know that he likes to believe it is behind us. It is hard for him to know how to think about it, how to be supportive. Is he supposed to think about dying in the middle of the night as do I? Is he supposed to join in my suffering each time I find a small new lesion? Should he face his mortality as I do? At some time, he will have his own chance. Right now I am just glad that we can sit across from each other at a restaurant, exchange stories, plan, dream, and create narratives that converge and sometimes go their own way.

April 12, 1989

Today I interviewed a woman lawyer for a study that I am doing on gender differences in professional ethics. When I began this research, I assumed that the interviews would mainly focus on the traditionally-defined ethical problems that lawyers face in their law practice: for example, confidentiality, conflicts of interest, and candor. Yet I am finding that most of the women I interview tend not to define ethics in those terms and instead see legal ethics as more global than I would have expected: for one lawyer, it was helping women; for another, it was empowering the disadvantaged. Ethical considerations appear to be at the core of their lives, a lens through which they see themselves and their work.

April 14, 1989

I just heard from Carolyn Harmon, my stepsister, that her husband Larry's cancer surgery went well. This is a relief. Recently, Larry was diagnosed with colon cancer and just two years ago developed thyroid cancer. Although Larry lived downwind from the Nevada Test Range, I am not aware that anyone attributes his cancers to this fact. Still, I am certain he speculates about it. Unfortunately, his chemotherapy and radiation treatment will be more difficult than mine, with possibly more nausea, since the radiation will involve the intestines. Larry was smart to see the doctor immediately upon developing minor symptoms. So critical is early detection that it can easily make the difference between life or death.

I always have been consistent about self-examination, and there is no question that I have saved my own life. Even now, Dr. Byyny and I agree that he should examine me approximately every three months, not only to spot change but to give me peace of mind, so that I will not always be worrying about some lesion. Sometimes it is hard to distinguish a lump from flesh that is rolling over a rib from normal variation in breast texture, so both Dr. Byyny and I keep separate written records and diagrams of the examination findings, noting the location of a cyst and its size. On one occasion I marked the results of my exam on the back of one of my business cards that I had in my wallet and hoped I would not accidentally give the card to someone! Yet even after having breast cancer, I have to force myself to do monthly self-examinations. It's important, so I never miss, but it is hard knowing what I might find.

April 24, 1989

Yesterday I participated in a nursing symposium on aesthetics and caring. My presentation focused on the relationship between caring and art or aspects of empathy and imagination that are important to both domains and also to ethics. I noted how the arts can help nurses develop a moral vision and a caring vision, looking at their lives and the lives of others in new and different ways. Then I reviewed one of my favorite stories by Henry James, "The Real Thing," in which a studio artist becomes a failure because he hires two models who do not require him to exercise his imaginative or empathic powers. Finally, I used a magnificent passage from Charles Dickens' *Tale of Two Cities* which observes "that every human creature is constituted to be a profound mystery to every other . . . that every beating heart in the hundreds of thousands of breasts there, is, in some of its imaginings, a secret to the heart nearest it? Something of the awfulness, even of Death itself, is referable to this." Dickens' lines also have poignant meaning for the experience of cancer, and its sense of separateness and even remoteness that confounds knowledge of another person.

My friend, Maxine Greene, gave the keynote address and was excellent, as she always is. Our mutual friend, Mary Ann Shea, joined us for dinner and some chitchat about what we have been doing the past months.

April 26, 1989

Last night Gordon and I hosted a dinner and lecture at our home to recognize the official opening of the Center for Central American Studies at the University of Colorado. Some very distinguished guests attended, including the Foreign Attaché and the former President of Honduras, the latter being the individual who played the most significant role in writing his country's constitution. For the occasion, we exhibited pre-Columbian artifacts in our gallery, my favorite being a small, solid, gold frog, about two inches in length. It is at least six hundred years old but shines brightly with eyes that look like large commas, arms extending straight, and legs ready to spring, to break loose in a desperate jump.

April 27, 1989

Today I went to the Health Science Center for an exam by Dr. Byyny. He assured me that everything was fine, and yet I can't believe I have gone six months without having another biopsy. Leaving his office, I felt a fresh exuberance about being alive, a clean awareness of the day. The wind whipped hair across my eyes as I walked out of the hospital, the same way that the wind funneled down this street when I came here a year ago for radiation treatments with knots in my stomach. Thankfully, today I can look at the buds forming on the trees without the distraction of fear.

Last night Gordon took Rebekah to get her braces. Actually, she looks very nice with them—the top teeth have clear bands that are hardly noticeable. On the way home, she pulled down the car mirror and said, "Yuck, I look like a teenager."

May 2, 1989

Rebekah is home ill today with allergy problems or a bad cold. She was sleeping this morning, so I came into the office for a while. Soon I will phone and see how she is doing and then probably leave for home, stopping at Dairy Queen to get ice cream for her scratchy throat.

Instead of driving to the mall this morning, I took a quick walk around the two ponds by the law school. A few students were lying on blankets, studying, and sunning themselves in the spring day. Whenever there is a hint of a warm day, students quickly turn out in shorts and bathing suits, lounge on dorm balconies, prop themselves against buildings, sprawl on the grass. Radios blare and voices come from residence hall windows. I remember a day early this spring when the students were sunbathing, riding their bikes, and playing with Frisbees, and then within five hours the temperature dropped forty degrees. A blizzard covered my car with eight inches of snow, and I was caught totally by surprise, in thin suede shoes.

May 9, 1989
(first entry)

Today I have a fairly quiet schedule in the office, returning telephone calls, answering mail, reading background material for my research. I do need to leave at 3:15 P.M. for a doctor's appointment to have some symptoms checked. There is a new small lump that I am concerned about, but also I have been feeling extra tired. Probably I am overworked, but these maladies give rise to thoughts of cancer. Each new health concern prompts me to think about the course of my personal development. While I do believe that I have grown reconciled to cancer, every time I find a new cyst I feel like that black dot, the one I dreamed about, waiting to be dashed by a wave against the shoals. I know I talked of transformations earlier in my journal—how cancer has given me fresh, fine-tuned recognition of aspects of nature and higher meanings of family relationships—but it is clear that not all of the answers and comforts have been found.

May 9, 1989
(second entry)

Just a quick entry to report that my examination went well. Dr. Robinson thinks I am feeling scar tissue in my breast from previous surgeries. Tonight I plan to go to bed early with the hope of remedying my symptoms of fatigue.

May 18, 1989

Last night I went to Rebekah's soccer game. Quickly, I spotted her at the distant end of the field because she is taller than her fellow players and has a long, gliding gate that gracefully carries her across the grass. She played well, although I could tell that she hesitated before running headlong and kicking into the pack of girls. Her friend, Tim, sat on the sidelines and watched until her team, the Burbank Thunderbirds, chalked up a win. After the game, she was tired, hungry, and very grumpy. A pizza quickly reversed her disposition, and we were soon engaged in animated conversation, planning where we would go to shop for a few summer outfits because all last year's shorts and shoes are too small. Once in the store, I found a comfortable chair and watched legs under a dressing room curtain step up and down.

May 20, 1989

I just returned from the field by our house. About seven this evening I went out and walked through the new green. The late sun was at just the right angle to make rainbows and brighten the grass to a silky luster. Dandelions absorbed the light, holding together in clusters. All along the footpath I thought of lifelessness turning to life, how new grass edged its way up through the matted path.

May 23, 1989

Last night we hosted a dinner for President Ding, the President of the University of Beijing. In terms of protocol, the evening was a near disaster. Our staff members, who take charge of social events and usually do remarkable work, were over committed and insufficiently researched the menu or etiquette considerations. Consequently, the quality of the food was poor, security for the President and his party was inadequate, guests were improperly greeted, and Gordon did not follow the right form for the toast. In addition, a news reporter arrived in the middle of the dinner announcing that he had a scheduled interview with Mr. Ding. Then the reporter simply walked into the dining room and stood there, until finally I got up to see who he was and what he wanted. I was so distracted and on edge from the disruptions and blunderings that I could hardly converse with our guests.

On the minds of everyone there were the student demonstrations at the University of Beijing that have been the leading news headline. The visitors from China spoke supportively of their students and the democratic wave sweeping China. They talked of wide public approval of the movement and the courage of the young protesters.

After the entree, Gordon stood and said a few words about Mr. Ding and about our university's desire to enter into a mutually-supportive relationship with the University of Beijing. Next Mr. Ding rose and quietly talked, in beautiful English, about his university, its goals and challenges. He acknowledged the dramatic events that were occurring on his campus, although he was very noncommittal about taking a position. He invited Gordon and me to visit his university and to help establish a student, faculty, and staff exchange with the University of Colorado. Afterward, when I had a chance to talk with him alone, he said he had been a math professor who was essentially forced to be president, and that he would like to go back to his old job. I recognized fear in his voice.

May 25, 1989

All day I have been hearing news reports about protests in Tiananmen Square in Beijing. I think that Mr. Ding and his party may have returned to China by now, but I can't get them out of my mind. What is happening to them?

Tonight was one of those romantic, scheduled "date nights" for Gordon and I. But instead of going out to dinner, we went for a drive into the foothills and through a few Boulder neighborhoods that we had never seen. It was nice to get away and to talk. Neither of us mentioned the cancer, but only discussed our forthcoming Memorial Day trip to Salt Lake City, Rebekah's summer schedule, and how Gordon plans to handle a difficult programming problem that is on his desk. His style of making decisions is very different from mine: He quickly assesses a situation and almost intuits the correct response, whereas I am methodical, deliberate, and prefer to think through all possible ramifications. When I consider Gordon, Rebekah, and myself, and the distinct ways we function in the world, I wonder if people have natures which are centering mechanisms for their whole being.

May 29, 1989

Today is Memorial Day. We came to Salt Lake City to spend time with family and to support Gordon's mother, since the holiday would undoubtedly bring to her a few difficult memories. Soon after arriving, we visited the grave of Gordon's father to see the headstone that had been placed there and to leave a bouquet of coral, yellow, and white flowers in a metal cylinder. His mother is lonely, and sometimes when she is riding in the car I see her turn her head and silently cry. When Gordon and I had some free time, we also drove to the Salt Lake Cemetery, so that I could decorate my father's grave and those of my Grandmother and Grandfather Cannon. It took me awhile to find my father's headstone, but finally I spotted some names that my mother said were nearby. Lying flat at one end of a gentle mound of dry grass is a small, gray rectangular stone. In block letters is written "Keith Clinton Dutson, 1920–1955." The cemetery is in the foothills of the Wasatch Range and sits high, overlooking the Salt Lake Valley—a wide, expansive basin rimmed by mountains. As we drove away, we passed an elderly man standing by a headstone which bore the name of a woman. The sky was clear, a few robins sang, and I thought of my mother saying that my father wanted to be buried where airplanes would fly over his grave.

June 1, 1989

Two days ago Gordon, Rebekah, and I returned from our trip to Salt Lake City, and today I am sorting a few old pictures my mother let me remove from her photo album. For a long time I have been thinking that I do not have any photographs of my father, or even earlier pictures of my mother and brother. My mother's album is a black, rectangular binder filled with heavy black paper and mostly three-inch square black and white photographs. The front pages of the book were of Mother at about college age, where in several of the pictures, she stands with a group of girls who are dressed more or less alike: dresses with short skirts, fitting bodices, wide lapels, and puffed sleeves that reached midway down their upper-arms. Like many of her friends, Mother's hair is dark, shoulder-length, and ending in a turned-under roll similar to the shape of the bangs that curl back from her forehead. Several of the young women in these pictures have remained her friends ever since junior high when they called themselves the "Shine-L's," because their names all contained the letter _L_. There also are pictures of my father in his early twenties, a tall, handsome young man with a thin face and broad smile. Sometimes he stands with friends or Mother's cousins and other times alone with her. I leaf through the album, and soon there are wedding pictures: Mother holding a cascading white bouquet, standing in a long, flowing silk dress which pools onto the floor, father in a dark suit with his hand around her waist. It has been years since I have seen these pictures, but I don't remember my father and mother looking so young. Wedding scenes are followed by pictures of Mother leaving the hospital, turning her head away from the camera to look at the baby girl in her arms. Then, there are others of me at one and two years old, riding in a carriage, looking up at the camera blank-faced, mouth opened, or sitting on the porch step next to my doll, "Baby Blue Eyes," about to pull two candles off a birthday cake. Keith is there too, with toddler legs that were always in motion. Quickly, I slipped several of the photographs out of their silver-colored corner holders, leaving a note that I would return them after I had made copies. As I lifted the album back into the box, I noticed several photographs grouped in a white folder. They were proofs of a formal portrait, Mother and I sitting together while seven-year-old brother, Keith, stood behind us resting his hands on our shoulders. I wore the red and white gingham dress mother had made me for Easter. I wear that dress in another picture, one in which my father stands holding my hand.

ཟ༹ *The Light Around the Dark*

June 4, 1989

It has been raining all week, which is unusual for Boulder. Tonight when I kissed Rebekah goodnight, water was running so hard through the gutters that she rushed to get into bed to listen to the sound of droplets splashing against tile roof. In West Virginia, I loved the rain so much that I would leave our house or my office to drive through the rolling hills where I would watch the lightning flash and a veil of liquid enfold the purple rim of the Blue Ridge Mountains. When I held Rebekah in my arms just now, both of us straining to hear water moving, her face looking up at me, I felt adrift in splendor of the day.

June 6, 1989

This afternoon Rebekah and I visited the Optical Electronics Laboratory of University of Colorado Professor Kristina Johnson. Kristina is a brilliant young scientist who is pioneering the development of a laser-based computer system. Because female students who are interested in science have few role models to show them a viable career path in physics, astronomy, or chemistry, I thought it would be inspiring for Rebekah to meet Kristina. Kristina walked us through her laboratory where graduate students filtered green light through a series of lenses, and photons passed in several ways through a small square crystal. We both could tell that Kristina loves her work—her voice was exuberant and hands fully animated as she introduced us to her colleagues and explained her research. Eleven years ago, while in graduate school, Kristina had cancer. The doctors said that it had spread throughout her body and that she did not have much hope of living. Shortly after I developed cancer, she told me of her experience with the red radiation line on her neck, one almost like mine, how the cancer, once so present, is now an exhausted nightmare. I look at Kristina, her vibrancy and assurance, and feel a sense of personal hope about my own challenge.

June 16, 1989

When Gordon came home tonight, he said that University of Colorado contacts with the federal government think that one or more people who were at our home for dinner with officials from the University of Beijing—just a few days before the Tiananmen Square Massacre—have been hanged. I look at the two embroidered silk boxes that rest on the shelf above where I now sit, gifts from President Ding, and I remember the look in his eyes when at dinner he rose to toast Gordon and the University of Colorado.

June 19, 1989

Yesterday Rebekah left for Computer Camp at Brigham Young University. Gordon is on his annual statewide summer tour. Today he is in Paonia and Montrose, and on Tuesday, Cortez and Durango. Every summer, Gordon spends three weeks visiting rural towns in Colorado, so that he can take the University of Colorado to citizens and let them see where their money is going. Gordon says this is the closest that he will ever come to a political campaign, what with local legislators, town leaders, new editors, speeches, handshakes, and barbecues—so many that Gordon turns green at the sight of baked beans. Usually, I protest his going, saying that he does not really need to go every summer, that it was good for a while but serves no measurable purpose to return year after year. Yet, I can tell by his voice when he phones me late at night that he likes to travel to small towns similar to the one where he was born and where there is the chance to visit down-to-earth, practical folk.

June 24, 1989

Rebekah is still at Computer Camp at Brigham Young University, and Gordon and I are enjoying a quiet evening to ourselves. We talked about us and how our lives have unquestionably changed, for the better, because of my cancer. Gordon, Rebekah, and I have had individual responses to the disease, and we have each taken private journeys. Sometimes I see Gordon sitting at his desk in the upstairs bedroom, closing his eyes, while other times he tries to talk about what it all means to him, how different he has come to feel about his work and family. But he says it is difficult to find words; this alone says a lot, because normally he expresses himself easily. Of course, Rebekah still asks a lot of questions: Will it come back? Did the doctors take out all the cancer? Are you feeling OK? She comes home from school and says one girl's mother has breast cancer, that it won't go away, that she is so sick. In Rebekah I can sense an undercurrent of anxiety, but there is also a strength and calm about her that is new. There has been a steadfast sense of peace with me, returning to the original forms that define my faith, my roots, and who I am— although I still have a long way to go in thinking about death and coping with health problems. Year after year, the recurrent lesions and surgeries are terrifying and make it difficult to put cancer in the past. Assuredly, life is a riddle. But I am not going to let go of this challenge, for I sense its importance, or its significance, in terms of my personal progression. A spiritual feeling tells me that whatever my problems may be, they are an intrinsic part of the abundance of life.

July 21, 1989

When going to bed last night, my eyes fell randomly on a medieval trunk that sits in front of the window. On top stands a four-inch high fairy, dressed in ribbons, blue butterflies, pearls, and a silver tiara. Overhead light filters through her transparent gold wings, their glimmer catching my eye. The hemline of the skirt of this little creature holds open a handwritten note from Rebekah for my birthday two years ago, which fell a day after my cancer surgery. It reads: "A Happy Birthday wish to my mom, With Love, Rebekah. Hope you like the present. I got it with my own money, I think you'll like this one better than the other one. You are the most wonderful mother that (here 'I ever' is crossed out) there is. I love you lots. Rebekah."

I have kept this memento in my bedroom since the surgery almost two years ago because it gives me a little boost every time the setting sun catches its wings, or its silhouette is drawn against the white shade. I think about how grateful I am to have this very daughter, what a wonder it is not only to see her become beautiful but to increase my understanding of how she grows, what inspires her, why she is able to read science fiction for hours when I fall asleep within the first five pages. She is like art that calls me to search its patterns and animating force, to explore her lines, her forms.

July 28, 1989

This morning, before heading off in our different directions, Gordon and I walked together through the neighborhood and around the Thunderbird Park pond, which is at the end of our street. The sun enhanced the blue of the sky and brilliantly lit the mountains and trees while the air's rare, cool vintage made the morning extremely lovely and glorious—the kind of beauty that is remembered and that stays with your perception as some kind of serene influence for a long time. We headed along a sidewalk that weaved through a common green area behind several homes, but we ran into a large snarling dog and quickly changed the direction of our route. Gordon and I are both terribly afraid of big dogs because when we were first married and living in a basement apartment in Yonkers, New York, Gordon was bitten on the neck by the landlord's mean dog. It was the day before his law school finals, and he had taken a break from studying to play Ping-Pong with the landlord's children. As he stooped to pick up a stray ball, the dog lunged at him, clamping its jaws onto his neck. I remember Gordon walking into our apartment, holding a bloody towel to his neck and calmly suggesting that we go to the hospital for some stitches. As it was, we spent most of the day in the emergency room, and Gordon still went to take his finals, although I have no idea how he managed to do so.

Thinking about the dog attack brings back memories of our newly-wed years living in that damp and cramped basement apartment. For several years, Gordon commuted to Columbia University every morning where he attended law school, and there I would board the subway for downtown and my first job, at the American Express Language Center. During this time, we shared a white Volkswagen Beetle that on extra cold days had to be rolled out of the driveway until it pointed down a steep street. Then Gordon would give it a good push and jump in next to me while I tried to pop the clutch. Finally, it would sputter into motion, and we would begin our drive through the backroads of Yonkers to avoid the first fifty cent toll on the Saw Mill River Parkway. At Columbia, the challenge was to find a parking place along streets lined two and three cars deep. Usually, Gordon found a space that no other car would dare try—sometimes with only two inches between our bumpers and those in front and back. At this time, his technique was to slowly move backward until the bumper gently tapped the car behind and then forward until we felt the front bumper tap, and so forth for ten or more tries.

Eventually, both the front and back bumpers of the Beetle became so concave that we could not open the hood or the trunk. At one point we tied a rope to the front bumper, then tied it to a tree, and gently drove back until something resembling the original contour was achieved.

August 14, 1989

This morning I went for a long walk in the field. Overhead, clouds with white frothy tops and gray bottoms spread widely across the vast panorama of blue. Now I can tell that autumn is coming by a fragrance of apples from nearby trees, the musty smell of dry grass, a gentle, cool breeze which blows hair into my eyes, and brown crickets jumping out of my way on the narrow dirt path. Today the field is thick with small white morning-glories, delicate blossoms with faces the size of quarters. They glow with the dawn's light which filters throughout the petals. Pink veins form a five-pointed star on the outer sides of petals and violet dots circle a yellow center from which tiny white stamens project. While some of the flowers are more heavily tinged with violet, and are of a variety that have been growing in the field since early summer, the clear white blossoms are new and seem to have appeared overnight. I pick a few, and they almost wilt as I watch—petals go limp, and the violet bloom closes in on itself. How do they manage to survive the dry, parched soil, the blazing sun, and yet fold into death so quickly when you break their tie to the earth?

August 26, 1989

Today is our wedding anniversary, and a card from Kitty Miller arrived as it has for the last twenty-two years. Ever since I was about five-years old, Kitty has been sending me greetings, first for birthdays but frequently now for our anniversary. On the inside of an old-fashioned floral cover—Kitty never sends slick new-style cards—

in her delicate, slanting handwriting is a brief, inspirational message that usually mentions God and life's blessings and then continues with a more lengthy summary of recent neighborhood activities. Since I have known her, she has lived in the same house on Twenty-third Street in Santa Monica, California. When Keith was two and I was five-years old, our family moved almost directly across from the Millers. Kitty's son Jack and I were in the same grade at school, and we quickly became best friends.

I spent many hours in Kitty's kitchen drinking milk and honey tea, tracing summer camping trips on the wall map, and hearing about her life as a young girl in Switzerland. Her hair was long and sometimes braided in a single strand that fell past her hips, although most times it was wound in a bun pinned at the back of her neck. As a young child, I thought of Kitty as extremely old, seeming more like Jack's grandmother than his mother, although she was probably in her early forties at the time. While it is true that children always think parents are old, I am sure my image of a frail, aged woman comes from her slender form which dipped painfully from side to side as she walked on a deteriorating hip socket. She was like my grandmother, someone who would comfort me, tell me stories about Switzerland, and have warm oatmeal cookies waiting after school

A year ago when Gordon, Rebekah, and I were on a brief excursion to Los Angeles, we drove past my old street because tracing and recording my personal history is now very important to me. I wanted to take a photograph of my childhood home and also one of Kitty's. We were running late for a plane and so made a brief stop, just time enough to jump out of the car and take some pictures. Surprisingly, the neighborhood looked pretty much the same as it did when I was ten, although my house and Kitty's seemed smaller than I remembered. Two years ago Keith visited Kitty. As for her house, he thought that nothing had changed since he played there as a five-year-old: the furniture, photographs, paintings of the Swiss Alps, the small square blackboard positioned at a child's height in the kitchen. Even the same paper map—absent of interstate roadways—was attached to the kitchen wall. And in the garage sat a red American Flyer wagon, the one Keith and I pulled with our oversized tricycle.

September 6, 1989

Rebekah is now getting into a regular school routine. She begins the day with choir and concludes with P.E., which are two good bookends that allow her an easy transition from home to school and from school to home. It feels good to get back into the autumn pattern, and a comforting and secure sense of order has returned to our lives. When summer arrives, I feel as though someone changes my psychological software and switches my internal word processing system from Word-Perfect to Microsoft Word, throwing me into a sort of chaos. With the end of the public school year, the more rigorous routine is stored for future use. And now as it comes again, I welcome it for the order it forces on the day.

September 15, 1989

Today is my forty-fourth birthday and also the second anniversary of my cancer surgery. This afternoon we are having a reception for several hundred new faculty at our home, but I arrived late because I stopped on the way home to have some personal time for reflection. I drove to a quiet, secluded spot close to the field by our home and read the personal journal I have kept for the past two years. Then I dictated some thoughts as an immediate reaction to the entries. Once in awhile, I tape-record my experience because I think it is important that family histories contain audio as well as written records. Gratefully, my Cannon grandparents recorded part of their family history. Shortly after receiving the tapes from my mother, twenty years after my grandparents' death, I played one in the car while driving to my office. I had not heard their voices since they were alive, and the memories they evoked of thin arms filled with snowballs and lavender and yellow iris, and strong but wrinkled hands bearing glass bottles of milk to the kitchen from the porch swelled over me like the morning flooding the field grass with sun.

I spoke into my small recorder about how I have been feeling: a certain sense of completion and fulfillment about new life challenges that began two years ago. Many of my goals are now accomplished: I regularly write in my journal, walk every day, pray often, set aside time on most days to read a little poetry or Scripture. Though it's hard to find time, I engage in more charity work, stay closer to friends, and monitor my professional work, so that I feel it more closely aims at the public good. Now I allow myself time to think about my personal philosophy and write about spiritual or life experiences.

Rarely is a day neglected aesthetically: I notice the subtle shades of green in the foliage around the law school pond, hear a gray finch calling its mate. And, too, I am newly aware of the yellow lacquer on a pencil, the glaze of a teacup handle, the soft texture of a brown sandwich bread. The September nights settle into piano chords, kisses on the corners of Rebekah's and Gordon's mouths, the smell of burned Parmesan cheese in the toaster oven. Sometimes Rebekah lets me lie next to her when she is going to sleep, and as I lie on my back dozing a bit, looking at the glow-in-the-dark solar system glued to her ceiling, I sense the close proximity of mortal and immortal life. I see windows opening to eternity, and I realize that this instant is everything. The day is not just movement from project to project or idea to idea, but rather is concentrated with subtle, profound life. Every moment holds everything.

September 18, 1989

Today we hosted a luncheon for Carlos Fuentes, the South American writer. He presented me with an autographed copy of his recently published book, *Christopher Unborn*. I took a few minutes to peruse the pages and was stuck by the narrator's voice: the voice of an unborn child. It was a haunting noise, the sound of a child on its way to earth. As I read, the child almost cast a glow of its form on the white pages. Then, late last night when I was straightening the kitchen, faces of hungry children paraded across the television: featureless mouths, blank eyes fixed on the camera lens, until my own reflection passed in the black glass of the microwave oven.

September 19, 1989

During my routine self-examination today, I discovered a lesion that seemed larger than the tiny grain-sized nodule I noticed a month ago. Finding these lumps happens so often that I almost feel I should not bother Gordon with the news. While he would want to know and would be sympathetic, I often feel like a complaining child who cries at the smallest hurt, who has not learned to signal parents about what is serious and what is not. When Rebekah was very young and would fuss every day about a stomach ache, or sore throat, or not feeling well, I would tell her that she must be more selective in her protestations, so that I could more accurately determine when she should see a doctor. Sometimes I feel as if Gordon would like to say: "Don't bother me with another false alarm; just let me know when it's cancer."

Of course, Gordon's admonition comes not from him but from somewhere deep inside me, from that source of nightmares that are now haunting my sleep: visions of my surgeon standing over me, Dr. Robinson looking grave as he tells me that the cancer has metastasized, my left breast collapsing and sinking into a well at the top of my rib cage. I'm so scared.

I think it is my fault if the cancer has returned, that I should have taken better care of myself: adhered to a low-fat diet, reduced stress, had more sleep. Health and wellness are not just about reconciling myself to having cancer, or even dying, it is a way of life that requires vigilance and discipline, a profound respect for the complexity and equilibrium of the human organism. Good health means diligence, control—more than I have. It's strange to me that the specter of death often does not provide sufficient motivation to effect change. In fact, I used to wonder how a friend diagnosed with lung cancer could continue chain smoking.

September 20, 1989

I am about to leave for Dr. Robinson's office. For a while I have been at work, trying to read and write—but I can't concentrate. A prickling sensation is creeping across my shoulders and down my arms, and the tips of my fingers feel cold. Under my ribs, a darkness seems to swell, moving through my abdomen, pulling, rolling, hooking like teeth into muscles, then plowing through nerves, turning up unseen dreams, memories: anesthetic odor, blood, pain, more waiting. I stare at the computer terminal and see myself walking along a steep precipice, one like the donkey trail at Bryce Canyon that I rode as a young child. Soon I will start feeling tired, exhausted, sleepy, as if all I want to do is lie down on the bedroom floor with my head on a small lace pillow.

September 21, 1989

Yesterday Dr. Robinson and Dr. Byyny both said they thought the new lump in my right breast had enlarged slightly since my last visit with them a month ago. Dr. Robinson performed an unsuccessful aspiration and an inconclusive needle biopsy, so now we are starting the wait-and-see game that I have played for the last twenty years, waiting to know if this is the beginning of the end.

September 22, 1989

When I got up this morning, I felt rested and happy but then remembered the biopsy that I will probably face soon. So difficult is it to live with fear and uncertainty, that all today I have been seeking some answer to or a deliverance from my despair. I do feel different and more at peace than I have in past years. And, too, I have learned something about moving beyond dread and anxiety, not only enduring hardships and accepting fate but seeing life as an affirming experience transforming pain into a love for life, including a love—almost—for the suffering that life means. In the television interview series, "The Power of Myth," Joseph Campbell talks with Bill Moyers about suffering, reminding us that the great myths say suffering is part of the lived life. However, he suggests that it is possible to achieve a state of mind in which the individual is rescued from fear and sorrow, moving beyond despair to an experience of rapture or even bliss.

This point of view was evident in a passage of Scripture that I read this morning in the *Book of Mormon*. The Scripture focuses on one of the main characters in the book, a young man named Nephi. Nephi's father, Lehi, a prophet and leader of a religious community, had just died. Two rebellious older brothers threaten to kill the younger Nephi. In a soliloquy on the occasion of his father's death, Nephi starts talking to himself: he wonders how to get beyond the wretchedness that he is suffering. I can almost see Nephi, sitting by his father's side, trying to kill the pain. The rain is falling, and he smells the blend of dust and vegetation which cling to the earth. There is little to say. He watches his father's hand fall back, and holds onto it, wondering where he is right now, if he is between worlds. He is aware of the space that once held his soul—Lehi, his father—that man who kept on going no matter what.

So Nephi goes to God, like a solitary echo. And then Nephi's soul starts rebuilding, remaking itself. It comes to him now, despair is transformed to joy, and he falls through pain, breaking out as a mud dauber wasp emerging from its cocoon where the imprint of suffering, broken-wing fragments, are embedded in a gold case. So it seems the story of life, what it means to be human, is necessarily paradoxical, for it finds life in dying, hope in despair, constancy in change, and great purposes in small means. It is as Campbell says: ". . . at the bottom of the abyss comes the voice of salvation. . . . At the darkest moment comes the light."

September 26, 1989

Surgery to remove the new lesions in my breast has been scheduled for next week. Normally I would be nervous, but an extraordinary thing happened this morning. I was in the parking lot, having just purchased breakfast, watching the morning sun fall on the Flatiron rocks and three small clouds turn almost crimson. I was thinking about Nephi and what Joseph Campbell said about the affirming conversion that suffering might yield, knowing that this should be my goal, when a powerful moment of illumination took hold of me. Suddenly, I felt a release from fear, from my fixation on biopsies, surgeries, and procedures. A blissful, rapturous quiet that cannot be put into words came over me. This, I know, was what Grandma Cannon meant in her journal in writing, "I almost felt happy," when bitterly crying in the outdoor latrine as her mother lay dying and her father knelt in desperate prayer. Her state of mind transcended to an ecstatic level that freed her from fear and despair. Grandma never forgot the moment: where she was, what she was wearing, what she was thinking, how she had descended into the dark, and abyss of suffering and hopelessness, and how suddenly she was swallowed by a new energy and radiance pulling her through the agony to where whole rivers of silk-like joy surrounded her.

September 27, 1989

I cannot get my mind off what occurred yesterday morning. I have not told Gordon or anyone else and do not know if I should or even could: language is so limiting. I fear talking about it or even that writing about it in my journal might make it appear trivial. I know my immediate reaction is to doubt when people say that they have had some type of spiritual or supernatural experience, except in the case of my grandmother who would never lie about anything or even exaggerate. I keep wondering what provoked my experience, that thrill of joy—if it was because I finally saw what might be attainable. Now I feel no heaviness of mind, no fear about the biopsy that will happen in a couple of days, no apprehension about waiting for lab results, no concern for the outcome of the surgery. The storm is behind me. Instead of despairing, I look out on the long expanse of my life to fine threads of light coming from all sides, to traveling through dark spaces but passing through to clearings.

October 2, 1989
(first entry)

My attitude about the approaching surgery remains true to my good feelings of this past week. Gordon, on the other hand, is eating full pints of Haagen Dazs ice cream and calling Dr. Robinson with new questions every day. "You're sure relaxed about this one," he observes.

Rebekah is auditioning for the play, _The Miracle Worker._ She has almost memorized the lines for every part in the script and has watched the Patty Duke and Anne Bancroft film version numerous times. When rehearsing the Helen Keller role, with eyes closed and arms swinging, she knocks objects off the kitchen counters or stumbles over the dogs. She has become very good at the part.

October 2, 1989
(second entry)

I had to write in my journal again today. A few minutes ago I returned from my lunch break. Each day I am trying to remember to take a few moments to experience being alive, to walk outside and take notice of nature, or simply to comprehend the afternoon. Today I walked around the duck pond by the law school. Saturday morning a severe windstorm blew branches, leaves, over-ripe crab apples, and pieces of bark into the water. From a distance the pond appeared covered with wood shavings, a golden mash through which ducks pushed, leaving ribbons of clear water in their wake. Across the bridge, where the storm's debris accumulated on the channel below, was a kind of mosaic of orange, gold, red, and little flames of yellow and green leaves shone bright in the afternoon sun.

October 4, 1989

The notation on my calendar says "11:00 A.M., Health Sciences Center," meaning when I should be at the University Hospital Clinic for the biopsy.

I finally told Gordon about what happened a few days ago, the spiritual experience, if you want to call it that, the elation. He had already noticed the change. "You became so peaceful," he said. Now I sit at the computer, waiting for Gordon to drive home to get me. I look out the window onto the field.

October 5, 1989

The biopsy is over. The procedure was pretty much the same as all others: Dr. Ketch performed the operation, removing a great deal of tissue through an incision less than a centimeter long—he hates scars—while Dr. Robinson and Dr. Byyny assisted and visited with me. I felt sorry for Gordon who had to stay in the hall by himself, but he did not have to wait long. The operation went quickly, and soon we were all engaged in conversation about matters having nothing to do with the procedure. Within a few minutes, Dr. Ketch received a call from the pathologist who reported that the cyst was benign. We all cheered at the good news, chatted a bit more, and then went our separate ways. All through the day, I never once felt fear, anxiety, or anything but a relaxed assurance, a subtle shifting of thought to Rebekah, Gordon, and geese moving blackly across the sky.

ࣿ *Epilogue*

October 9, 1990

Breckenridge. I have been in our mountain home in Colorado for two days now, trying to put finishing touches on a manuscript that represents two years of my personal journal entries. It snowed all day yesterday, setting records for snowfall and low temperatures. The first storm of the winter is always invigorating, and I feel a quiet, exquisite zeal that I remember from my childhood, a state of pleasant emotion that carries with it an acute awareness of physical sensation. There was a tenseness in my shoulders as I watched the flakes take their long route to the ground, first blowing horizontally above the pines before starting a downward spiral into the branches and onto the clearings of grass. This morning the sky is completely clear, blue, unbelievably vivid and beautiful. Mounds of snow hang from tall, slender pines, a slight breeze pushing them back and forth or lifting and lowering their weighted branches. Once in awhile a gust blows a lump of white from the pine needles, creating a small cloud of fine crystals. Bach's *Mass in B Minor* is playing on the stereo, the Franklin Stove is radiating a comforting warmth, and fresh mountain air blows through a small crack in the window across the table from where I work.

It is almost a year to the day since I have had problems with my breast or a biopsy of any kind. Although all medical tests have indicated no new cancer or metastasis, two weeks ago I did discover another lump. Because of my heavy work and travel schedule, I could not immediately run to Dr. Robinson.

I can't help thinking about cancer. When I found this new spot under my arm, I was filled with fear. A panic gripped my stomach muscles and stiffened my neck. A dark film seemed to envelop every thought, and I felt that I was falling into another world. Where was that peace, that assurance, that I felt I had so mastered? The faces of young women I have known who did not recover from breast cancer— Nancy, Stella, Jan, Dorothy, Betty—found my dreams, and I awoke with my breast throbbing and shooting pain.

But soon enough the fear started to surrender to that peaceful reassurance, and it is with me now, a sense that I am in touch with something higher than myself, or something higher within myself—an understanding. I feel that I am connecting again to those spiritual frameworks that turn suffering toward joy. I must work with them. But this may mean that I am gaining my own control of such feelings as opposed to having them hit me almost as a gift.

On my drive up to the mountains to our home, I stopped at Georgetown, an old mining town that is very beautiful in the fall. Around the small town park are yellow aspen and birch which stand against a white Victorian band shell and wood-sided, pastel homes. I pulled the car to the side of the road and watched leaves blow in circles. A little whirlwind moved on the dirt road, sweeping twigs, pebbles, and soil into a miniature frenzy. I thought how I wanted again to touch that source that turns sorrow to delight.

I just returned now from outside where I sat in the sunshine, surrounded by snow-ladened pines, watching the stream flow into the pond. A single opening in the sky held glimmering crystals, grass protruding up through the snow, a chipmunk chattering in 4/4 time, and delicate tones of wind chimes from a house across the road.

Intermezzo

❧ *A Daughter's Tribute*

My mother is with us today and will be forever. I love her very much and miss her more than I can convey to you. Perhaps I miss her so much because she had three roles in my life—my mother, my sister, and my best friend. We always said we grew up together.

So my loss is that much greater. When I think of my mother and her legacy, a number of words come to my mind: courage, grace, dignity, faith, love, strength, a sense of humor, intelligence, humility, compassion, giving, caring and—to the last day—an incredible love of life.

Mom had wonderful courage. When she was very ill, we always called it "Eskimo courage." We called it that because we had gone to a movie about Cole Porter and hairy men, dressed in Eskimo suits, sang. One day when Mom was getting a chemo treatment, I said, "Mom, remember the Eskimo men." She laughed and from then on when we would do our "Jane Fonda" (our daily exercises), we would use our Eskimo courage. In her last weeks she was very bloated. She had a lot of fluid in her body, because her heart wasn't working, and we'd hear her little fat feet thump around the hall and her voice saying, "Eskimo courage." Her main goal was to be there for my 16th birthday. During my birthday party she came downstairs. It was the first time she had done that in months, and as she walked up the stairs I could hear her saying "Eskimo courage."

Mom had great faith. She loved her Heavenly Mother and Father very much. Before we found out about her recurrence of cancer, we were flying on the airplane together, and she heard a voice that said "Something is going to happen, but everything will be all right." Through her illness she always referred to that and said, "Rebekah, no matter what happens, I'll be there for you and everything will be OK."

She had a great love for women. She was very concerned about issues of race and gender and also very concerned for other people who had cancer. She loved Dad and me very much and always called me her "Heaven on Earth." She wrote songs for me and would always say, "Sweetest girl in the whole wide world" in her melodic voice. The night before she died, she told the nurse how much she loved us and the last thing she said to me was how much she loved me.

She had a great sense of humor, a wonderful smile, and a quick wit. She'd always say witty things that you wouldn't think were funny at first until you thought about them for a while and then they were really funny. When we were in England, we were on the bus to Windsor Castle, and she wanted to get off the bus. She said, "This is the Windsor Castle stop," and I said, "No it's not, Mom." We got out and were standing in front of a big building. (As it turned out, Windsor Castle was about 30 miles away.) She asked the bus driver, "Is this Windsor Castle?" Everybody on the bus roared with laughter. Mom thought it was hilarious, too. I was mortified.

She had great compassion and loved to help people. She helped one of my good friends, Kelly Larson, to get through school. Mom was so proud of her and was helping to pay for her to get through graduate school when she died. Kelly recently adopted a baby and Mom was so proud. They named her Lindsey Elizabeth after Mom.

Another really good example of her compassion was a family she helped in Colorado. They were going through hard times, and the children were not getting the support that they needed. She would go to their house almost every day and bring them flowers and toys and give them hugs and tell them she loved them. She helped them to believe in themselves. They moved to Arizona and are doing a lot better. Their oldest daughter often used to call Mom for support. Mom really changed their lives around by caring about them.

She was very humble. She was a beautiful woman and had a beautiful spirit. She was extremely bright, and I'd always tell her so, and she would laugh at that. She never thought that she was really beautiful or intelligent.

She was very giving. She always encouraged people to reach their full potentials. A few days before she died she wrote to a dear friend, Mary Ann Shea, "I hope you can reach your goals, and I'd like to help you reach them." I think this statement really represents her.

Finally, she had a great love of life. On the day before she died, she wrote to her friend, Maxine Greene, "Maxine, I'm going to keep on fighting. I don't know for how long, but I love life and its small joys and the delicate patterns of the holly leaves."

It made her happy just to walk outside and look up at the trees. In the fall she was really scared one time and went out for a walk. She saw a beautiful tree, with its leaves turning red and gold, and looked up at the branches and saw how they interacted with the sky. She said she felt a sense of peace because she loved nature and everything that Heavenly Father created.

I love her very much, she is my greatest kindred spirit and she will always be with me.

Rebekah Elizabeth Gee

For Elizabeth

A song of
     sun filtering through lace curtains
     high tea with cucumber sandwiches
     scones and lemon curd
     or herbal tea and scraped apples

A song of walking
     through pampas grass
     around the Oval
     up and down rows of book stacks

A song of scholarly pursuits
    through qualitative methodology
    professional discourse
    and weaving in parallel themes from literature

A song of kindred spirits—
    Maxine Greene
    Mary Ann Shea
    Marilyn Krysl
    Phyllis Updike

A song of travel
    Breckenridge
    New York
    London
    Moscow

A song of leadership for women
    West Virginia
    Colorado
    Ohio

Mary M. Davis

These remarks were given at Elizabeth D. Gee's funeral by her daughter, Rebekah.

Coda

In late October, Elizabeth called from her room at University Hospital in Denver and asked if I would please come be with her. I remembered her visit to our South Carolina home the previous June when she had asked me to be with her in her dying time and speak at her funeral, and I had responded that I would honor that, but also wanted to share her living time. I felt she had now arrived at the intersecting point of living/dying.

When I arrived at the hospital from the airport, I navigated through security by using her maiden name, and went to her room. Many of Elizabeth and Gordon's personal things I recognized, but the bed was empty. It was a sunny, crisp autumn day and I thought perhaps Gordon had taken her out for a brief walk. The assumption was in vain and it quickly took a nosedive as I learned she was in ICU. My heart sank with sadness as I sensed what was unfolding. Gordon met me in the hall with his usual affable greeting but this time coupled with an uncharacteristically stern voice, "We need to talk before you see her." We did. Then we went in to see her. She appeared to be asleep, but the atrial fibrillation and cardiac monitor witnessed to the 200 beats per minute, and the struggle of the jugular vessels, surging against the neck of her gown. Her cardiovascular system was clearly compromised. I wondered if her heart space was fighting with the same intensity. Her jaundice was distressing, too. Gordon turned to me and said, "Well, what do you think? She's pretty damned sick, isn't she?" Elizabeth then opened her eyes, and with an audible sigh, "Oh, I'm so glad you're here."

One morning after I had read to her, we had some private time and she asked if I would bring her Bible to her. I laid a pillow over her legs and opened the Bible on top. She took the precious yellow baby blanket of Rebekah's and rolled it up under her head and began reading the entire chapter of *Proverbs 31* —one of her favorites. She paused when her eyes would not focus, or when she wanted to share the meaning of a special verse with me. She never faltered at the myriad of frustrations, as if some inner boundary was negotiating its own path. I felt reverent toward her tenacity and insistence on giving something to me and told her so. This woman and dear friend was heroic, indeed, and was offering many gifts even in the midst of her serious illness.

We reminisced about our many and varied times together and how we felt we had become sisters. We felt that way soon after we had first realized that the dates of our birth were only fourteen days apart. We talked of our husbands, our children, our longing to make contributions to the world, the blessings, fears, challenges and delights in balancing many selves into one. She confided that she was ready for a miracle but also prepared to die. I remembered our conversation the previous summer by the lake when she said she could "see" five years ahead—to Rebekah's college days—and felt confident she would be there for those events.

October 28th was the day scheduled for her radioactive monoclonal antibody treatment. We talked of it being my son's birthday and a hope of new life for her. Gordon, her mother and dad, and I carefully prepared the room where she would receive her treatment. Rebekah's presence was always keenly felt. Elizabeth asked me to transfer her photographs to the other room—the same room where she was hospitalized after her bilateral mastectomy four years earlier. An unsettling association. There were lovely personal photos of Rebekah, of Rebekah and Gordon, of special occasions. I carefully made rolls of masking tape beneath each picture on a nearby wall so she could see them with ease.

The next part I have chosen to share with great difficulty as the memory moves from the realm of privacy to public. Elizabeth was deeply committed to the notion that the health sciences at the cutting edge blended with aesthetic and personal care values. It is my conviction that she advanced both, and received both. One experience was scholarly; the other was lived in the flesh and spirit. At her request, I bathed her before her treatment and then smoothed on one of her favorite lotions. I fought back my own tears and rage as I knelt down and massaged her edematous toes, arches, and feet—the footsteps that had travelled so far—geographically and metaphorically. I gently massaged her back around all the tubes—port of entry into a body—and a life. She sighed as her shoulders released their tension and said how wonderful it felt. I managed a small portion of comfort myself in staying with her suffering and admitting to myself the portion of suffering that was mine.

The "silver bullet" arrived from nuclear medicine. People called in from the hall and announced everything was in order and they were ready for Elizabeth. The time was now—the excitement and hope was palpable. Elizabeth said she would like Gordon to say a blessing before the treatment began.

Gordon came to her side and held her as we encircled her bed with clasped hands—her husband, her daughter in spirit, her mother and father, and myself. I was especially touched by Gordon's offering of Thanksgiving, which preceded requests for healing. We each gave her a quick hug. The reality of not being allowed to touch her during and after the treatment seemed to be an alienating counterpoint to what had just transpired.

We sat side by side in her window sill and watched as the first golden drops released from the drip chambers. The team watched as the nuclear physicist waved the golden Gieger counter over and above Elizabeth and then around the I.V. tubing to monitor the emission of radioactivity. Did he really make the sign of the cross in the air? Or was it my need and projection to see an embodied expression of the priest(ess)/healer?

An hour and half later, she sat up in bed and ate most of a regular meal. The metatases in her substernal area, her lungs, her liver continued to challenge her mindbodyspirit. She was heroic in her efforts always. The next day we could touch each other if there was clothing between us to absorb the radiation. She took my arm as we walked in the hall with her portable oxygen tank. When we reached the west windows, she asked to stop and marvel at the breathtaking view of the snow-covered front range.

Many humans struggle with the question, "Is there life after death?" I would propose that there is an equally powerful and critical question that all of humanity must address first, and that is: "Is there life after birth?" Elizabeth addressed this question magnificently with her very being. Sometimes I think about humans existing as embodied spirits during this time we presently know as our lifetime. In other words, the body/physical may be the gift of divine clothing. Martha Graham spoke of our bodies as sacred garments, our bodies being sacred garments in that we are born in them, live in them, and are required to honor them. On December 17th, in early morning, Elizabeth left this garment and moved more fully toward the sacred. I think of her presence especially at dawn, perhaps because she often feared the shadows which preceded it.

Last year, I was privileged to go to Haiti as an invited international health consultant. Elizabeth said she would love to be able to go with me. The magnitude of pain and suffering of Haitians is immense and at times overwhelming. However, every day at five o'clock in the morning, we were awakened by singing outside our windows. With every fiber of my being, I believe that Elizabeth has now joined those whose Song of Life announces the movement from darkness to light at dawn. In closing, I give thanksgiving for the love and life of Elizabeth Dutson Gee that we have been privileged to share. A gift, indeed, of the highest order.

Amen

Phyllis Updike, RN, DNS
Associate Professor
School of Nursing
University of South Carolina